THE · BUSINESS · SIDE · OF · GENERAL · PRACTICE

# The Law and General Practice

EDITED BY
DAVID PICKERSGILL

RADCLIFFE MEDICAL PRESS
OXFORD

British Library Cataloguing-in-Publication Data
A catalogue record for this book is available from the British Library

ISBN 1-870905-57-1

Phototypeset by Intype, London
Printed and bound in Great Britain by
Biddles Ltd, Guildford and King's Lynn

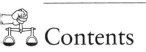 Contents

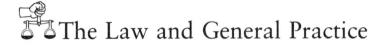

The Law and General Practice

Contributors

LYNNE ABBESS, *Hempsons, Solicitors*

KATHLEEN ALLSOPP, *Deputy Chief Executive, The Medical Defence Union*

JOHN BURTON, *HM Coroner for Greater London and Honorary Secretary, Coroner's Society for England and Wales*

NORMAN ELLIS, *Under Secretary, Contract Services Division, British Medical Association*

GARETH EMRYS-JONES, *Chairman, Rural Practices Subcommittee, General Medical Services Committee*

JOHN FRY, *former Member of Council, Royal College of General Practitioners*

JEAN HARRIS HENDRIKS, *Consultant Psychiatrist, Child and Family Service, Dunstable*

EDWARD JOSSE, *Regional Adviser in General Practice, North East Thames Region and Associate Dean of Postgraduate Medicine, British Postgraduate Medical Foundation*

DAVID MCLAY, *Chief Medical Officer, Strathclyde Police*

HELEN PHILCOX, *Brown, Muir, Mackintosh and Co., Solicitors*

GERARD PANTING, *Secretary, Medical Protection Society*

JOHN OLDROYD, *Secretary, Secretariat for London Local Medical Committees*

ALAN ROWE, *Consultant, European Health Affairs*

RALPH SHIPWAY, *Le Brasseurs, Solicitors*

DAVID WILLIAMS, *former Chairman of the Statutes and Regulations Subcommittee, General Medical Services Committee*

RICHARD WILLIAMS, *Consultant Psychiatrist, Royal Hospital for Sick Children, Bristol*

Editor

DAVID PICKERSGILL, *Chairman of the Statutes and Regulations Subcommittee of the General Medical Services Committee, British Medical Assocation*

The Business Side of General Practice

Editorial Board

Preface

THE relationship between the law and general practice is much closer than many general practitioners (GPs) might at first realize. All GPs will be aware that the services they provide for their patients are governed by their Terms and Conditions of Service, which in turn are enshrined in the NHS Acts. However, many other aspects of the law have an important bearing on the doctor's ability to practise. Not only do doctors have to relate to their patients, but they increasingly have to deal with third parties who are anxious to obtain information about patients registered with individual GPs. The doctor must be aware of the constraints which the law places on him in responding to these various requests.

This book does not seek to be an authoritative textbook on the law but sets out to provide an informed discussion of the various aspects of the law with which every GP should be familiar and an understanding of those laws which will make successful practise so much easier. For more detailed information, the reader may wish to consult the original Acts, or take advice from their own solicitor or defence society.

DAVID PICKERSGILL
May 1992

Acknowledgements

I am extremely grateful to all the contributors for their chapters. They are all experts in their own fields and have produced their contributions with enthusiasm and worked to a very tight timescale. I would like to thank *General Practitioner* for their kind permission to reproduce an original article by Richard Williams and Jean Harris Hendriks.

I am deeply indebted to my secretary, Mrs Gillian Kemp, who has retyped many of the original manuscripts after editing and amendments.

The members of the Editorial Board have been enormously helpful in providing extensive comments and suggestions for inclusion in the book and I thank them.

Finally, my work on the General Medical Services Committee (GMSC), which has enabled me to develop my interest in the law and general practice, would not be possible without the help and support of all my partners and in particular, my wife, Hilary. I am very grateful to them for their help and support over many years.

1   Partnership Agreements

Lynne Abbess

Types of partnership

THE definition of a partnership is found in Section 1 of the Partnership Act 1890 which states: '*Partnership is the relation which subsists between persons carrying on a business in common with a view of profit*'.

The Act provides for the establishment of what is commonly known as a 'partnership at will' which imposes all the obligations and liabilities of a partnership upon its respective members without building in any safeguards. Thus it is possible for any one partner to serve notice to dissolve the partnership at any time and without giving any reason.

The purpose of a partnership agreement is to supplement the provisions of the 1890 Act, which is lacking in modern commercial reality, so as to provide a secure working base for all parties. However a partnership can be established merely by the parties coming together and declaring that they are practising together as partners; there does not have to be a formal partnership agreement. Because of the NHS regulations governing medical partnerships it is often considered necessary for the partnership to be established before the parties know each other. As this working relationship is often compared with that of marriage this might be rather foolhardy! To overcome this difficulty it is recommended that partners take on a prospective partner as an assistant in the first instance with a view to partnership. Although this is likely to incur expenditure for the existing partners which may not be reimbursed it is considered a prudent safeguard. As an alternative, a partnership agreement may be entered into *before* a new partner joins the practice. This contains a probationary period which allows either side an escape mechanism within the probationary period. The worst scenario is to allow a doctor to join the practice as a partner on day one without any form of agreement as this will leave the original partners very exposed.

Why have a partnership agreement?

A 'partnership at will' can be brought to an end just as easily as it is formed. There is no requirement in the 1890 Act for there to be any justification for such a decision and although the Act does not permit expulsion, in circumstances where a majority of the partners wish to get rid of one particular individual the partnership can be dissolved by any one of them and then reformed as a new partnership immediately afterwards, thus providing no protection for any individual within the group.

The effect of dissolution (particularly immediate dissolution) can be devastating for the following reasons.

Surgery premises

With the dissolution of a partnership any partner who does not have an interest in the surgery premises will face exclusion from those premises. Usually it is possible to argue that such a partner, who would be termed a 'licensee', should have not less than 3 months in which to vacate the premises. However this is a short time in which to find, acquire and set up suitable new premises which are acceptable to the doctor concerned, the FHSA, the local planning authority and the patients.

Jointly owned premises also present difficulties as they will have been structured to accommodate one practice only and the division of the partnership will create at least two practices. It should be remembered that the partnership is separate from the joint ownership of the premises and the fact that one partner may have decided to end the partnership does not give him any greater right to occupy the surgery premises than other joint owners. Ultimately any joint owner of the premises has the right to seek a court order that the property be sold under Section 30 of the Law of Property Act 1925. This however would be a last resort as the cost of making such an application could run to tens of thousands of pounds and does not guarantee that the party making the application will be entitled to buy the premises.

Restrictive covenant

Unless it has been expressly agreed and documented there will be nothing to prevent any partner from setting up in competition with the remaining partners. Thus should one partner elect to dissolve the partnership he may be set up in competition next door (subject to planning consent and FHSA approval etc) or even within the same premises in the event of him jointly owning them. Now that it is easier for patients to move from doctor to doctor this is likely to cause even greater problems than in the past.

Continuation election

Unless there is a declaration requiring each partner to do so there would be no obligation on any one partner to sign a continuation election for Inland Revenue and tax assessment purposes. Without such an election the business of the partnership would be deemed to come to an end with effect from the Notice of Dissolution and a new business would commence, thereby exposing the partners to the opening and closing rules. In most cases this would produce severe and adverse tax consequences for the partners.

Problems

In addition to the problems created by the dissolution it should also be remembered that unless declared to the contrary the Partnership Act implies that each partner receives an equal share of the profits. Furthermore there would be no provisions relating to agreements for holiday entitlement, sickness entitlement, etc. Thus if a partner were on sick leave he would be entitled to continue to draw his full share of the profits whilst the other partners cover for him and the cost of any locum tenens would be a partnership expense rather than an individual expense for the duration of such leave.

Without a partnership agreement individual partners are severely exposed.

Where to go for advice

The British Medical Association (BMA) issue a booklet on partnerships and the GMSC have recently published a revised checklist of 10 essential points which should be included in a partnership agreement together with an explanatory note containing further proposals.

Family Health Services Authorities (FHSAs) may discuss criteria with you, although the role of the FHSA is geared towards the protection of patients rather than the individual doctor. The Secretary of the Local Medical Committee will usually be prepared to offer advice, and should be able to provide the names of appropriate experts if further advice is required.

In order to prepare a partnership agreement it is important to take proper legal advice from a solicitor with the relevant experience. A solicitor may be experienced in the principles of non-medical partnerships but unless he is aware of the implications of the NHS Regulations and the 'Red Book' he will be unable to advise you adequately.

In the event of a dispute, the content of a partnership agreement will be analysed and, regardless of its title, construed on its content. In a recent case a deed entitled 'partnership agreement' was analysed as being no more than a contract of employment as a result of which the FHSA sought to reclaim £46 000 worth of allowances paid to the equity partners of the practice. This situation had arisen because the deed had been prepared by a solicitor friend of the partners who had no knowledge of medical partnerships. Any costs incurred in producing a properly drawn deed will be considerably less than the costs of resolving a dispute at a later date.

What areas should the partnership agreement cover?

1 Parties names and addresses.
2 Commencement date.
3 Declaration relating to termination of the partnership.
4 Capital assets

- sale and purchase of shares
- time scale and provision for interest
- valuation methods with particular reference to Cost Rent Schemes.

5 Occupation of premises by non-owning partners.
6 Expenses: individual and partnership.
7 Income: individual and partnership with particular consideration being given to notional/cost rent income.

8 Schedule of profit shares from commencement date to parity.
9 Partners' obligations to each other.
10 Partnership accounts

- drawings
- tax reserve
- year end
- accountants

11 superannuation.
12 Holidays and study leave.
13 Sickness and maternity entitlement.
14 Retirement: voluntary and compulsory.
15 Effect of retirement or death – restrictive covenant.
16 Arbitration provisions.
17 Declaration re patients.

It is essential to include all aspects of your particular practice. It may be that certain minor aspects will change in which case it will be possible to provide reference within the agreement to the existence of a separate document which may be revised without the need to go through the formalities of changing the partnership agreement itself on every occasion. Any variation in the future should be carefully documented and minuted and the minutes themselves initialled by all those concerned.

Rights of individual partners

Under the 1890 Act it is assumed that all partners have equal rights. There may be some variation within a partnership agreement but the rights of individual partners should not vary too greatly lest doubt might be cast as to whether the relationship is one of partnership or more realistically one of employer and employee. Thus rights to take holidays, etc. should all be equal. The main exclusion to this rule would be a variation in profit shares leading to parity, although it is generally accepted that parity should be achieved in no more than 3 years. Any variation in hours worked can of course be reflected in profit shares subject always to the 'one third/one quarter/one fifth rule'.

The decision-making process within partnerships

Generally a partnership should distinguish between day to day matters and policy matters. The latter would include decisions on the admission or expulsion of a partner, variation in profit shares, new premises, etc. Usually the former decisions would require a majority only and the latter would require a unanimous decision. In larger partnerships however it may be unworkable to require unanimity on every decision, in which case, a greater than 50% majority may be required, e.g. in a partnership of six partners an 80% majority may be required which means that the decision of five partners will carry the vote. Clearly any decision relating to a specific partner will be made on the basis that that partner does not have a vote. Thus if there is a suggestion that one of the six partners should be expelled an 80% majority would allow four out of five partners to carry the vote (the sixth being excluded from the vote).

In case it may not be immediately apparent whether a decision should be one of policy or one of day-to-day routine, an additional clause could be incorporated within the agreement, allowing a preliminary vote to be taken to determine the matter, the majority required to be e.g. 65% thus allowing four out of six partners to carry the vote.

Consideration should also be given as to whether it is essential for all partners of the practice to be present for a decision to be taken, whether proxy votes are to be permitted and how a matter should be dealt with in the event of an equality of voting. Previously it has been considered acceptable for the senior partner present to have a casting vote but these days it is considered inequitable for one partner to have greater rights than another and accordingly it will be usual to provide that the *status quo ante* should prevail.

Intervals for review of the agreement

It is essential that the agreement is kept under constant review so that changes can be recorded. There is no particular time-scale for this but partners should certainly reconsider their deed on each of the following events:

1 the retirement or death of a partner (the deed will normally provide what should happen in such circumstances but there might be other

changes made within the partnership as a result of this which should be recorded);

2 the admission of a new partner;
3 any changes of working patterns within the partnership regardless of the change in the identity of the partners;
4 the acquisition or disposal of premises;
5 any further changes in the Regulations;
6 the effect of any case law (this would normally be reported in the medical press)
7 any variation to the practice area.

It should be stressed that none of the above may result in the need for a new deed but consideration should be given as to the way in which any of these affect the existing partnership structure and relationship as recorded in the partnership agreement.

Mechanisms for settling review

Depending upon the extent of the variation required, the matter can be dealt with in a number of ways which ultimately reflect the weight of evidence required in the event of a subsequent dispute.

Record in the partnership minutes

As in every business it is essential that regular meetings are held and minutes recorded. This method of review could cover the situation where agreement is being reached pursuant to the terms of the original partnership agreement, e.g. the partnership agreement says that a partner may hold an outside appointment with the consent of the other partners and provided it does not interfere with his duties to the partnership. If an individual partner puts forward details of such an appointment which the other partners consent to it should be recorded in the minutes and initialled by each of the partners as evidence.

Supplemental partnership deed

Typically this covers the position of an incoming partner to the practice where the main terms of the agreement have not changed but it is necessary to record:

1 the identity of the new partner;
2 any probationary period
3 the revised profit sharing schedule.

Revised partnership agreement

This would be necessary where a radical review of the partnership structure has taken place. Many partnerships who have had an agreement drawn up which is now out of date may consider it prudent to have an entirely new deed rather than to have a long supplemental partnership deed which may be more difficult to interpret. Similarly partnerships who have had a succession of changes within the partnership and thus a succession of supplemental partnership deeds may consider it advisable to start afresh on the admission of the next new partner.

Advice to incoming partners

It is essential to settle the terms of partnership *before* admission. At the very least you should ensure that you receive an offer of partnership setting out the essential terms of the agreement which should be acceptable to you and in an ideal world you should be presented with the form of the existing partnership agreement and should enter into a supplemental partnership agreement so that all parties know where they stand before the new partnership commences.

If you have serious concern about any aspect of the partnership before entering it do not be fooled into thinking that matters will improve following your entry. An established partnership is unlikely to be willing to change merely to meet your demands. You would be better off reserving your position and seeking an alternative partnership whose members are more in tune with your way of thinking.

You would be advised to take accountancy and legal advice on the 'deal' presented to you. Any legal advice that you take on the terms of a partnership agreement should form a partnership expense rather than your own individual expense. It has been suggested that if a new partner is denied this opportunity he may be entitled to argue in the future that he was effectively press-ganged into signing an agreement which he did not understand (although it may not be wise to rely on this argument and it would certainly be safer to seek proper advice!).

You should consider particularly your prospective security in the new partnership; this will be reflected in part by the number of patients you are offered on your list and your ability to purchase a share in the surgery premises (if these are privately owned by the partners).

Advice to remaining/outgoing partners prior to change

The most important point to remember here is that judicial opinion now supports the school of thought which proposes that a partnership deed will only be binding on the partnership if **all** members are party to it. Failing this it is suggested that such a partnership deed would not be binding on **any** of the parties. This means that your hard work in negotiating the terms of a partnership deed in the past will come to nothing unless you ensure that a new partner will be bound by similar terms. Evidence of this would be required, the best evidence being a further partnership deed (usually referred to as a supplemental partnership deed). Failing this, at the very least, there should be evidence that an offer of partnership has been made to a prospective new candidate on the basis that he is prepared to be bound by the terms of the existing agreement even if a supplemental agreement at that stage has not been entered into. It would be prudent to attach a copy of the existing partnership agreement to any offer of partnership so that there can be no doubt about the precise terms on offer.

It will be apparent from the above that if a partnership agreement is not entered into the existing partners can be severely exposed. Obviously the mirror image of all that has been stated under the preceding heading should be taken into account although it is fair to point out that the position of the outgoing partner may be different from that of the remaining partners.

Partnership premises

In the case of an incoming partner replacing an outgoing partner it would be easy to assume that the incoming partner should purchase the outgoing partner's share in the premises. However this may not provide the best solution for the remaining partners. An outgoing partner should be entitled to payment of his share within 12 months of the date of retirement to enable him to benefit from Capital Gains

Tax retirement relief. However, it may not be prudent to require an incoming partner to purchase such a share if it falls within his probationary period. This may 'squeeze' the remaining partners but it should be considered a preferable alternative to the problems that could otherwise arise.

Generally the advice to all partners in the event of a change in the structure of the partnership is **be prepared** so that matters are not rushed at the last minute when hasty decisions might have to be made.

Maternity leave and partnership agreements

The combination of the fact that the Sex Discrimination Act 1975 now applies to partnership of all sizes (previously it applied to partnerships of 6 or more) and various European Court decisions has effected a change in the way in which maternity leave is considered within a partnership context. It is now necessary to show that a female partner receives no lesser benefit for maternity leave than either she or her male partners would receive on sickness leave. This relates both to the length of the leave available and to the financial benefits available. Thus in a partnership where the partners agree to cover the absence of a partner on grounds of sickness for e.g. 28 days in any calendar year and provided a female partner is given not less than 28 days maternity leave without expense the partnership will not be in breach of the sex discrimination legislation. Indeed it would be usual to grant a female partner more generous rights and now that FHSAs reimburse locum costs for up to 13 weeks this is usually regarded as a starting point and the GMSC explanatory notes record this. (Remember that the FHSA reimbursement may be less than the actual cost of providing a locum tenens.)

Problems occur in circumstances where partners elect to effect insurance at the partnership expense against the cost of providing a locum tenens to cover any individual partner's sickness for e.g. up to one year. In these circumstances a female partner would be entitled to similar terms for maternity leave. The answer to this problem may be to allow each partner to effect his own individual locum policy at his own expense which would provide him with similar cover on grounds of sickness but which would not present the same difficulties with regard to maternity leave.

Judgment of 'reasonable' behaviour

This should normally be an objective test, i.e. how would the reasonable man (or as Lord Denning has said, 'the man on the Clapham Omnibus') judge the behaviour of an individual partner, although it should also be judged in the context of that specific partnership. It is easy to cite obvious examples of what would be considered unreasonable, e.g. stealing, but there are far too many points to recite here in respect of the less obvious cases. In order to determine the position, professional advice should be sought, and unless the decision is clear cut partners should not take hasty action which may prove embarrassing or impossible to substantiate in the future.

Methods of valuation of assets

This can be divided into two types of assets: premises and assets within the premises, ie fixtures and fittings and equipment, etc.

Premises

General

Normally a partnership agreement would provide that each partner be entitled to appoint a valuer to assess the value of the premises in the hope that the respective valuers can then agree a valuation. In the event of disagreement, provision should be made for a third valuer to be appointed with the agreement of both valuers, whose decision should be final and binding.

Consideration then needs to be given as to the basis of valuation. Usually this will be on the basis of a willing buyer and a willing seller in the open market with vacant possession (although there may be variations required depending on the particular circumstances of the case, e.g. if part of the premises owned by the partners has been let to a pharmacist, part of the property will be considered to have an investment value). Further consideration should be given as to whether or not there should be a deemed restrictive covenant affecting the property, limiting its use to that of a doctors' surgery only. Failure to incorporate this would allow a valuer to take into account any prospective development value the site may have, or alternative uses which may be attributable to it (e.g. office use) which may impose a higher value. As rent reimbursement is assessed on the value of the property as a doctors' surgery this could create difficulty for the remaining partners.

Ultimately the sum to be paid to an outgoing partner, or the sum paid by an incoming partner, will be the value of that partner's share of the equity in the property, i.e. that partner's share of the capital value less any outstanding mortgage.

Cost rent scheme

It is essential in cost rent schemes for an agreement to be entered into at the same time as the acquisition of the property or of an individual partner's share of the property. The agreement should provide that the value of the property should be either the value of the original cost of purchase and development or the value of the share as set out above, whichever is the greater. Thus, on the occasion of a change in the property ownership, in circumstances where the value has not caught up with, and overtaken, the original cost an incoming/outgoing partner will neither be required to inject any capital nor receive any (the only exception to this rule being that in the case of a repayment mortgage a small amount of capital might have been paid back in which case the partner's share of that value will be payable/receivable). However, failure to agree such a deed could result in an outgoing partner being required to pay back his share of the outstanding loan which exceeds the current market valuation of the property. In view of the fact that continuing partners are likely to continue to receive the full cost rent reimbursement this is considered unfair. Do not be caught out by thinking you are protected, or that there is a general agreement within the partnership to this effect, because if there is nothing in writing you will have an uphill struggle to prove your case.

Other assets

There are two alternatives in these circumstances. Either the assets can be independently valued on the open market (as above) or the written down book value can be taken. Generally, partnerships are structured on the basis that an incoming partner will be required to put in a sum of working capital which will incorporate his purchase of a share of these assets on the written down book value, but advice should be sought as to the basis proposed, prior to a commitment being made.

2 Employment Law

Norman Ellis

Introduction

WITHIN the confines of a single chapter it is only possible to summarize the key features of employment law. Reference should be made to other sources for a fuller explanation of the law and its implications for GPs.[1]

As employers, GPs are subject to an extensive range of employment legislation. Over the past 25 years, some 16 Acts of Parliament have been implemented establishing over 20 new legal rights for individual employees (*see* Figure 2.1). This plethora of legislation has been enacted by successive governments to encourage a more formal and equitable approach to industrial relations and personnel matters. Other influences on this legislation have included comparisons with established international standards (e.g. the Equal Pay Act and Sex Discrimination Act, and impending European legislation on part-time employment) and legislation in other fields such as the Race Relations Act. Although this body of employment law is intended to alter the personnel policies of all organizations, irrespective of size, the special position of the small employer whose circumstances and resources are greatly different from those of the large organization has often been ignored by legislators. There are some important concessions to size (most of which have been recently implemented); but the totality of employment law does impose a significantly greater administrative burden on a small employer.

The overriding aim of any employer should be to avoid litigation. This can be achieved by good management practice, including taking a more formal approach to many employment matters.

The remainder of this chapter summarizes key aspects of employment legislation in these areas:

[1]See Ellis N (1991) *Employing staff*. BMA, London

Individual rights	Eligibility (length of service)	Principal legislation
To be given a minimum period of notice – based on length of service – of termination of employment	1 month	Employment Protection (Consolidation) Act 1978
To be given written particulars of terms of employment	Immediately* (the employer has 13 weeks in which to supply it)	
To receive equal pay with a member of the opposite sex doing similar work	Immediately	Equal Pay Act 1970
Not to be discriminated against on the grounds of marriage or sex	Any stage from advertising of job	Sex Discrimination Act 1975
Not to be discriminated against on the grounds of colour, race, nationality, or ethnic or national origins	Any stage from advertising of job	Race Relations Act 1976
Not to be unfairly dismissed	2 years*†	Employment Protection (Consolidation) Act 1978 and Employment Act 1980
To receive a guaranteed payment when no work is available	1 month*	
To receive payment when suspended on medical grounds – in certain specified industries only	1 month	Employment Protection (Consolidation) Act 1978
Not to be dismissed on pregnancy grounds	2 years or immediately if regarded as sex discrimination	
To receive payment for absence due to pregnancy or maternity	26 weeks	Social Security Act 1986
To return to work after absence due to pregnancy or maternity leave	2 years	
Not to have action – short of dismissal – taken against him/her because of trade union membership or activity	Immediately	
To have time off – with pay – for carrying out trade union duties or for approved industrial relations training, if trade union is recognised for collective bargaining purposes	Immediately	
To have time off for trade union activities if trade union is recognised for collective bargaining purposes	Immediately	Employment Protection (Consolidation) Act 1978
To have time off for public duties	Immediately	
To have time off – with pay – to seek alternative work or to arrange training if made redundant	2 years*	

To have protection in case of employer's insolvency	Immediately	
To receive an itemised pay statement	Immediately	Employment Act 1988
To receive on request a written statement of the reason for dismissal	2 years	
To have paid time off for antenatal care	Immediately	Employment Act 1980
To have a protected period of notice and for his or her trade union – where recognised by his or her employer for collective bargaining purposes – to be consulted if made redundant	Immediately	Employment Protection Act 1975

* Employees working 16 hours or more a week are eligible. After 5 years' continuous employment, employees working 8 hours or more a week are eligible.
† If dismissal is for certain inadmissible reasons – that is, for reasons of trade union membership or activities – there is no length of service qualification.

Figure 2.1: Individual employment rights. *Source:* Ellis N (1991) *Employing Staff*, BMA, London

1 the employment contract: what it should contain and how it can be changed;
2 statutory sick pay;
3 statutory maternity pay;
4 health and safety in the surgery;
5 disciplinary and dismissal procedures;
6 redundancy;
7 discrimination;
8 part-time employees.

The employment contract

A contract of employment exists as soon as an employee shows his or her acceptance of any employer's terms and conditions of employment by starting work, and both employer and employee are bound by the terms offered and accepted. Often the initial agreement is verbal not written, but within 13 weeks of an employee starting work the employer is legally obliged to provide a written statement detailing the main terms of employment with an additional note on disciplinary procedures. (This requirement does not cover staff who normally work fewer than 16 hours a week, unless they have worked for 8 or more hours a week for 5 years.)

This statement must contain the following information:

1 names of parties to the contract;
2 date employment began and statement about continuity of employment.
3 job title;
4 pay;
5 hours of work;
6 holiday entitlement and holiday pay;
7 sick pay;
8 pension;
9 notice of termination;
10 grievance, disciplinary and appeals procedure. (Employers with less than 20 employees are exempt from including information on the disciplinary procedure.)

It is sensible to prepare and issue a comprehensive contract of employment that covers all these subjects. (BMA members can obtain a model contract of employment from BMA regional offices.)

Attention paid to preparing a correct contract of employment ensures that unforeseen and unwanted disputes do not arise. The preparation and agreement of the contract should ensure that the employer is reasonably familiar with his or her legal responsibility and obligations and has not unknowingly acted contrary to these at the outset. Moreover, if any dispute should arise and a GP has to defend personnel practices and policies, the doctor's position is greatly strengthened if it can be shown that he or she acted in good faith and had taken reasonable steps to act in accordance with the law.

The statutory requirement to provide written statements on these matters does not have to be supplemented in any way. There is no legal obligation to provide a written contract as such. But in practice the written statement of the main particulars of employment (together with your policy statement on health and safety matters) can be regarded as the basis of a written contract of employment. The contract as a whole also includes the job description (whether written or not) and the many informal and undocumented understandings and working practices which always form an important part of any employment contract. An example of these informal and unwritten practices are the arrangements normally followed when staff take coffee and tea breaks, including allocating the duty of making coffee or tea for the GP and his or her partners.

Changing a contract

A written contract may have to be changed; no difficulties should arise if a correct procedure is adopted and the substantive reason for the change is 'reasonable'. There are several approaches to changing a contract and the key principle underlying these is that an employee should normally consent to any changes before these can become contractually binding, irrespective of whether this consent is implied or by express agreement, given in advance of or at the time of the change.

Obviously, an employer should seek to reach agreement on the proposed changes. If consent is obtained this can either be given by express agreement, orally or preferably in writing. In any case, an employer is required to put in writing the terms of the contract (as changed) if it relates to any of those subjects listed (*see* page 16).

Alternatively, consent may be shown by implied agreement which is normally assumed if an employee continues to work under the new contractual terms without complaint.

The written contract itself may contain provisions that allow for changes in matters such as pay, the place of work, working hours and the duties of the job. Nevertheless, even if a contract is drafted broadly in this way, an employer must be prepared to show that the change itself is reasonable and was implemented in a reasonable and fair manner.

If consent is not forthcoming, even though the employer has made considerable efforts to agree the change with his or her staff, implementation on a unilateral basis requires a reasonable period of notice. Normally, any contractual change imposed by an employer without an employee's consent will be a breach of contract. If this is a fundamental breach of contract, hitting at the heart of the contract, an employee may be entitled to claim compensation for unfair dismissal. But by giving sufficient notice of the change, normally at least as long as the notice required to terminate the contract, it may be possible to avoid these problems. Even if this length of notice is given, the employer could still be liable to pay compensation for unfair dismissal or redundancy. The advantage of giving adequate notice of the change is that the employee is likely to be left with little or no time to protest after the change is actually introduced.

In summary, the reasonableness of any change to a contract of employment is subject to both a procedural test and a substantive test: two questions have to be addressed:

1 has the employer proceeded in a reasonable way by seeking agreement and giving adequate notice?
2 is the proposed change in itself a reasonable one to want to make in the particular circumstances of the business?

Statutory sick pay

The statutory sick pay (SSP) scheme establishes a minimum entitlement for sick pay for most employees. Every employer is required to pay sickness benefit as the agent of the government, but the decision on whether sick pay should be paid lies primarily with the employer rather than the Department of Social Security (DSS).

The main features of SSP are:

1 National insurance (NI) sickness benefit is no longer payable for most sickness absence; instead SSP is paid directly by the employer;
2 SSP is paid in the same way as normal pay and is liable to deductions for income tax and NI contributions;
3 entitlement to sick pay does not depend on previous NI contributions or previous service with the employer;
4 married women paying the reduced contribution and part-timers are entitled to SSP provided that their earnings are above a specified figure;
5 the total SSP that may be received from one employer for one or more periods of sickness cannot exceed 28 weeks' worth; after 28 weeks state benefit may be claimed from the DSS;
6 the employer has to decide whether sick pay is payable;
7 the employer can deduct the amount paid out in SSP from remittances to the Inland Revenue of NI contribution, although no deduction can be made for any amounts paid in error;
8 SSP is paid at three rates according to the average weekly earnings of the employee.

The rules of SSP are quite complicated and need to be applied correctly. Every GP should have a free copy of the DSS's booklet *Employers' Guide to Statutory Sick Pay*.

Statutory maternity rights

Most practices employ only a small number of staff but the majority of these are women. The employment rights of the expectant mother are intricate and stringent. Thus, any employer with a small number of staff may be faced with serious administrative problems if a member of staff becomes pregnant.

An expectant mother does not have a right to maternity leave as such; in fact, she can acquire four distinct employment rights:

1 not to be reasonably refused paid time off work for antenatal care – applicable to all employees irrespective of their length of service;
2 to receive statutory maternity pay (SMP) if she has 26 weeks' recent continuous employment with an employer and normal weekly earnings above the NI lower limit;

3 to complain of unfair dismissal if dismissed because of pregnancy;
4 to return to work with her employer after a period of absence on
account of pregnancy and confinement.

The last two rights are acquired by an employee only if she has been
continuously employed for at least 2 years and normally works for 16
or more hours a week, or for at least 5 years if she normally works
for 8 to 16 hours a week. But great caution is advised if an employer
is contemplating dismissing a pregnant employee who has not acquired
these specific employment rights.

This area of employment law is most complex for employer and
employee. It is vital that any GP should obtain detailed guidance on
how to ensure an employee obtains her statutory maternity rights. The
DSS has published a free booklet, *Employer's Guide to Statutory
Maternity Pay*; every GP should obtain a copy of it. Any mistake,
even if it is due to ignorance or a misunderstanding of the law, could
lead to a tribunal case and costly compensatory award. Industrial
tribunals are assiduous in upholding the rights of pregnant employees
and impose severe penalties in cases where unfair dismissals have
occurred because of pregnancy.

Health and safety in the surgery

The Health and Safety at Work Act 1974 requires an employer, including a self-employed person, to provide and maintain a safe working
environment, and it has established powers and penalties to enforce
safety laws. The main thrust of the Act is to make both employer and
employees more conscious of the need for safety in all aspects of the
working environment. The most important duties are those that any
employer must fulfil to staff, i.e. all that is reasonably practicable
to ensure their well-being. The words 'reasonably practicable' are
important; what is expected of an employer depends on the size of
the business and the resources available. Thus, in general practice, a
larger partnership carries a heavier burden of responsibility than one
that has fewer staff and resources.

The law requires an employer to provide information, training and
supervision for staff on health and safety matters. Unless there are
fewer than five staff, the employer must provide a written statement

of general policy on health and safety arrangements for implementing this. It can be included in the written contract of employment.

The GP also has a duty to ensure the safety of anyone who enters the surgery or health centre, including patients, visitors, building contractors, tradesmen and health authority staff. If the premises are owned by a private landlord or a health authority, the licence or lease may impose this duty upon these other parties and they may also be liable if there is an accident.

Disciplinary and dismissal procedures

An employer is required to include details (or specify where these are to be found) of his or her disciplinary procedure and the rules governing an appeal against disciplinary action. (Employers with fewer than 20 employees are exempted from this requirement.) Disciplinary rules and procedures should promote fairness and order in the treatment of individuals. They also help a practice to run effectively by setting standards of conduct and performance at work and ensuring that these are adhered to, and also by providing a fair method of dealing with alleged failures to observe them. Disciplinary procedures should not be seen primarily as a means of imposing sanctions; their main purpose is to emphasize and encourage improvements in individual conduct and performance.

With effective disciplinary procedures, and also effective selection and training procedures, dismissal should be a very rare occurrence. In general, employees who have not completed 2 years' continuous employment by the date on which a dismissal takes place, or who work fewer than 16 hours a week unless they have been employed continuously for at least 8 hours a week for more than 5 years, cannot complain of unfair dismissal. This also applies to employees who have reached the normal retirement age for their employment or, if there is none, men who have reached 65 years or women who have reached 60 years.

The risk of a successful claim of unfair dismissal (which can involve compensation payments of many thousands of pounds) can be largely avoided if the procedure adopted is both fair and reasonable, and the reasons for the dismissal are also fair and reasonable. An employer may have to justify his or her actions so it is wise to keep detailed documentation throughout. Finally, any BMA member contemplating a dismissal, but who is uncertain about how to approach it, should not hesitate to contact his or her BMA regional office for advice and assistance at the earliest possible opportunity.

Redundancy

Redundancy is still rare among practice staff, but it is becoming more commonplace as practices adjust to the demands of the 1990 contract. However, unfair dismissals on the pretext of redundancy are, regrettably, much more common; it is often thought that redundancy is a more acceptable way of getting rid of an unwanted employee.

When a redundancy occurs important legal obligations fall upon the employer. An employee has a statutory right to receive redundancy payments and paid time off from work to look for another job if he or she has at least 2 years' service and works at least 16 hours a week, or 5 years' service and works between 8 and 16 hours a week. These same qualifying conditions also determine whether the employee has the right to claim unfair dismissal if a redundancy selection has not been made fairly according to objective criteria.

Under employment legislation redundancy is defined as a dismissal caused by an employer's need to reduce the number of staff. Normally an identifiable area of work should have disappeared. A dismissal cannot be regarded as a redundancy if the employer immediately engages a direct replacement, but an employee with different skills or in a different location may be engaged (unless the redundant employee could be required under the contract of employment to work at the other location).

Normally any employee of a practice, when it changes hands, automatically becomes an employee of the 'successor' practice on the same terms and conditions. It is as if the employee's contract had originally been made with the new practice; continuity of employment is preserved, as are any rights acquired under the old contract. So when staff are transferred in this way no dismissal has occurred and thus there is no entitlement to a redundancy payment.

An employer must make a statutory lump sum redundancy payment to any employee with at least 2 years' continuous service who is dismissed because of redundancy. Self-employed people or members of a partnership do not qualify, neither do male employees over age 65 or female employees over age 60. Employees on fixed term contracts of at least 2 years' duration which include, with explicit written agreement, a clause waiving entitlement to redundancy payments are also disqualified.

The amount of the lump sum payments depends on how long the employee has been continuously employed, how these years of service relate to particular age bands, and on weekly pay (the current maximum in 1992 is £6150). An employee does not pay tax on a statutory redundancy payment but an employer may set it off against tax as a business expense.

As far as possible objective criteria, precisely defined and capable of being applied in an independent way, should be used when determining who is made redundant. This ensures that employees are not unfairly selected for redundancy. Examples of such criteria include length of service, attendance record, experience and capability. The chosen criteria must be applied consistently by any employer irrespective of the size of his undertaking, and the decision should normally reflect some combination of the above criteria.

Great care must be taken if a practice is considering making an employee redundant, otherwise it could be faced with a claim for compensation for an unfair dismissal. BMA members should contact their regional office at the earliest opportunity for expert advice on how to handle this difficult situation. Far too often redundancy has been used as a pretext for dismissing employees who are not in fact redundant. The consequences of using redundancy for the purpose of dismissing on grounds of inefficiency or incapacity, where there is no genuine redundancy, can be very serious indeed. A successful claim for unfair dismissal can require an employer to pay an employee a five figure sum as compensation. This compensation cannot be offset against taxation, nor can any part of it be reimbursed by the FHSA or Health Board.

Discrimination in employment

GPs rarely experience any difficulties with the race and sex discrimination laws. Of course, avoiding discrimination per se is good management practice. It may seem unlikely that a small business with only a small number of employees (most of whom are women) could be affected in any way. But both the Race Relations Act and the Sex Discrimination Act apply to all employers, irrespective of size. Previously the Sex Discrimination Act applied to all employers apart from those with 5 employees or fewer; recently the government introduced legislation which ended this exemption for the small employer.

There are two areas where legislation requires an employer to act (and to be able to show that he or she has acted) in a manner that is not discriminating:

1 on the grounds of sex (including equal pay) and marital status;
2 on the grounds of colour, race, nationality (including citizenship) or ethnic or national origins.

If a practice's recruitment and selection procedures, together with its employment practices, are properly conducted no difficulties should arise. Although sex discrimination legislation was intended primarily to improve the status and opportunities of women in employment, GPs, whose staff are almost wholly female, should note that men do have equal rights under this legislation.

The scope and structure of both the sex and racial discrimination laws are similar. Both include two types of discrimination, direct and indirect, and both require employers to take essentially the same action to ensure that their behaviour is neither discriminatory in practice nor capable of being seen as such.

Direct discrimination occurs when a person treats another person less favourably on grounds of race (or sex, or both) than he or she treats (or would treat) someone else. It is not necessary to show that the person openly expressed an intention to discriminate: it is possible in many instances to infer that the motive was discriminatory in the light of the circumstances of his or her actions.

Indirect discrimination occurs when the treatment may be equal in a formal sense but is discriminatory in its effects on one sex or particular racial group − for example, an unnecessary stipulation that a cleaner should have certain educational qualifications.

When assessing whether an employer has acted in an indirectly discriminatory manner an industrial tribunal is required to consider whether his or her actions, although formally applied in a non-discriminatory manner, have the effect of being discriminatory.

There are three areas where it is unlawful to discriminate on grounds of race or sex when recruiting staff:

1 in the arrangements for deciding who should be offered the job;
2 in relation to any terms of service offered;

3 by refusing or deliberately omitting to offer a person employment.

It is also unlawful for employers to discriminate on grounds of sex or race in the promotion or training opportunities they provide for their employees, and also in respect of any other benefits, facilities or services.

The most important matter on which a practice may need to concentrate is its arrangements for selecting and recruiting staff. The more informal its methods the greater the risk of being accused of discrimination, particularly on grounds of race. An approach based on 'word of mouth' methods can easily leave an employer open to a claim (even from someone unknown to the practice who has not actually applied for the vacancy) that the selection procedure is discriminatory.

Part-time staff

A large majority of practice staff are part-time. In general the part-time employee has fewer rights to employment protection than the full-time counterpart. But the law is quite precise about who is a part-time employee for the purposes of applying these rights and which rights are for all employees, irrespective of how many hours a week they work.

The law regarding all employees who work 16 or more hours a week and have 2 years' continuous service, and employees who work between 8 and 16 hours a week and have 5 years' continuous service, as qualifying for certain employment rights (these are summarized in Figure 2.1).

Employees working less than 8 hours a week have no claim to any of these employment rights. But certain other employment rights are universal and not dependent on the number of hours worked or length of service; these include rights under sex and race discrimination legislation, rights against victimization or discrimination for trade union activities; and rights to paid time off for antenatal care.

3   Statutes and Regulations

David Williams

Acts of Parliament (primary legislation)

An Act of Parliament consists of consecutively numbered paragraphs, called sections, which may be divided into numbered subsections. The Act may be divided into parts and the text may refer to schedules. Schedules are to be found at the end of the Act, are numbered and consist of consecutively numbered paragraphs and sub-paragraphs. Schedules, too, may be divided into parts.

An Act is usually preceded by an index headed, 'arrangement of sections', which indicates the purpose of each section, the division into parts and titles of the schedules. To become an Act, a parliamentary Bill must, normally, have received the approval of both Houses of Parliament together with the formality of the Royal Assent.

Statutory instruments (secondary legislation)

As parliamentary time is limited, Acts of Parliament are usually confined to the general intention of the legislation. Authority is given in the Act for the issue of secondary legislation (statutory instruments) to fill in the detail. Secondary legislation may be subject to parliamentary control. The statutory instrument may be required to be laid before the House or before both Houses either in draft form or after being made. To come, or to remain, in force, the statutory instrument may require:

1 affirmative resolution of one or both Houses; or
2 the absence of a negative resolution; or
3 no further action
  as specified in the Act authorizing the secondary legislation.

Statutory instruments may include orders-in-council, statutory regulations and statutory rules. Power to make statutory regulations and rules is usually given to a Secretary of State.

A statutory instrument will start by giving the dates on which it was made, laid and came into operation and will quote the Act and section under which it is made. It will consist of consecutively numbered paragraphs called regulations, rules, or for orders-in-council, articles. These may refer to schedules which will be numbered and are found at the end of the statutory instrument proper.

Reading and interpreting acts and statutory instruments

Every Act and statutory instrument adds to, amends or repeals existing law. It follows that the text may be altered by any subsequent Act or statutory instrument. A fully revised and accurate text incorporating all changes to date is essential. Usually, that is not available and this can be a major problem. Particular care is required in noting amendments and repeals and in reading the section (or regulation) governing the meaning of words used in the Act (or statutory instrument). For example, Section 36(5) of the National Health Service and Community Care Act 1990 is repealed by Schedule 10 of the Act itself.

Legislation may be confined to England and Wales or may extend to, or be confined to, Scotland and Northern Ireland. From time to time, legislation may be consolidated in a new Act.

The National Health Service Acts

Although the National Health Service was established by the 1946 Act and reorganized by the 1973 Reorganization Act, legislation was consolidated in the National Health Service Act 1977 and the National Health Service (Scotland) Act 1978. Subsequent legislation had relatively minor effect on general practice until 1990. The 1990 Act extensively amended the 1977 and 1978 Acts which cannot now be read without reference to the later amendments and repeals, and they have all been consolidated in the 1992 Act.

For general practice, the most relevant Acts and sections of those Acts are as follows.

National Health Service Act 1977

1 Consolidation.
2 General Medical Services (Sections 29–34). Definition of GMS (Section 29).

3 Pharmaceutical services and dispensing by doctors (Sections 41–43).
4 Local Medical Committees (Section 44).
5 NHS tribunal (Section 46–49 and Schedule 9).
6 Exercise of choice of practitioner in certain cases (Section 50).
7 Prohibition of sale of goodwill (Section 54 and Schedule 10).
8 Power of Secretary of State when services inadequate (Section 56).
9 Health Service Commissioner. Not to investigate GMS (Section 116 and Part 2 of Schedule 13).
10 Powers to make orders and regulations (Section 126).
11 Definitions (Sections 128).

National Health Service (Scotland) Act 1978

1 Consolidation.
2 Health Boards (Section 2). Constitution (Schedule 1).
3 Scottish MPC (Section 3). Membership (Schedule 2).
4 Local Medical Committees (Section 9).
5 Power to supply goods to practitioners (Section 15(1)).
6 General Medical Services (Sections 18–22).
7 Medical Practices Committee and distribution of doctors (Sections 23–24).
8 Pharmaceutical services and dispensing by doctors (Sections 27–28).
9 NHS tribunal and disqualification of practitioners (Sections 29–32).
10 Power of Secretary of State when services inadequate (Section 33).
11 Exercise of choice of practitioner in certain cases. (Section 34).
12 Prohibition of sale of goodwill (Section 35).
13 Residential and practice accommodation (Section 48).
14 Private practice by practitioners in health service accommodation and facilities (Section 64).
15 Charges for drugs, medicines and appliances (Section 69).
16 Remuneration of members of NHS bodies (Section 88).
17 Health Service Commissioner for Scotland (Sections 90–97). Not to investigate practitioners (Schedule 14).
18 Interpretation (Section 108).

Health Services Act 1980

1 Introduced District instead of Area Authorities in England and Wales with consequential amendments of the 1977 Act.
2 Amended Section 42 and 43 of the 1977 Act relating to the right of the patient to obtain drugs from a person of his choice (Section 21).

Health and Social Security Act 1984

1 Established Family Practitioner Committees as free-standing bodies independent of District Health Authorities (Section 5) with consequential amendments of the 1977 Act (Schedule 3).
2 Inserted a new Section 43A into the 1977 Act and a new Section 28A into the 1978 (Scotland) Act requiring the Secretary of State to make regulations providing for the remuneration of persons providing general medical services to be determined from time to time by 'such authority as may be specified'. (Section 7)
3 Amended Section 44 of the 1977 Act regarding Local Medical Committees (paragraph 7 of Schedule 3).

Health and Medicines Act 1988

1 Arranged the sale of the General Practice Finance Corporation (Sections 1–6).
2 Introduced retirement for GPs at 'an age specified in regulations' (Section 8).
3 Introduced abatement of pension for GPs re-employed after first retirement after the age of 65 years (Section 9).
4 Introduced explicit powers to investigate matters relating to general medical services whether arising on complaint or otherwise (Section 17).

National Health Service and Community Care Act 1990

1 Introduced Family Health Service Authorities (Section 2) and defined their membership (Part 2 of Schedule 1).
2 Defined the 'primary functions' of authorities (including FHSAs) and permitted them to provide similar services by entering into an NHS contract (Section 3).

3 Altered the constitution of Health Boards in Scotland (Section 27 and Schedule 5).

4 Defined an 'NHS Contract' (Section 4).

5 Amended Section 15 of the 1977 Act to redefine the duty of an FHSA; Section 17 of the 1977 Act to allow Regional Health Authorities to give directions to FHSAs; and further amended Section 44 of the 1977 Act to allow FHSAs (instead of the Secretary of State) to recognize local medical committees as representative and to allow them to delegate functions (Section 12, Section 29 for Scotland).

6 Provided for fund holding by practices (Sections 14–17, Section 34 for Scotland).

7 Introduced indicative amounts for drug budgets (Sections 18 and 35 [Scotland]).

8 Subjected the NHS to the Audit Commission (Section 20 and 36 [Scotland]).

9 Amended the 1977 Act in relation to the Medical Practices Committee allowing the Secretary of State to alter the constitution in the 1977 Act and to give directions (Section 22 and 38 [Scotland].

10 Allowed the Secretary of State to limit the total number of GPs; transferred, in circumstances to be prescribed, the power of selection from the Medical Practices Committee to the FHSA; and made new provisions for job sharing and appeals (Section 23 and 39[Scotland]).

11 Allowed an authorized registered medical practitioner to exercise powers of medical examination and of inspection of medical records in relation to certain premises in which community care services are being, or are proposed to be, provided (Section 48).

Consolidation Act 1992

National Health Service regulations

GPs ought to make themselves familiar with the NHS (General Medical and Pharmaceutical Services) Regulations 1974 and with the NHS (Service Committee and Tribunal) Regulations 1974 as amended to date. The regulations have been extensively amended and further amendments are issued quite frequently. The General Medical Services Committee of the BMA has issued an unofficial version of the NHS

(General Medical and Pharmaceutical Services) Regulations 1974 incorporating all amendments to July 1991. The Department of Health has issued an unofficial consolidated text of the NHS (Service Committee and Tribunal) Regulations 1974 as amended incorporating the Amendment Regulations 1990 but not the Amendment (No 2) Regulations 1990. These were part of the Notes of Guidance on complaints procedures issued to FHSAs. NHS GPs are entitled to a copy of the 1974 regulations with amendments on appointment and should receive further amendments as issued. Fund-holders may require the NHS (Fund Holding Practices) (Applications and Recognition) Regulations 1990. Parallel regulations have been issued in Scotland.

Statement of Fees and Allowances

This is also known as the Red Book. It is prepared under Regulation 34 of the NHS (General Medical and Pharmaceutical Services) Regulations 1974 as amended. Because it is prepared under Regulation 34, failure to comply with the Statement might, in certain circumstances, be construed as a breach of the Terms of Service. Failure to study the Red Book will almost certainly cause a doctor to lose fees and allowances to which he is entitled and to miss opportunities of practice development.

Terms of Service

These are contained in Schedule 2 of the NHS (General Medical Services) Regulations 1992 and the status of that schedule is defined in Regulation 3. However, it is very important to appreciate that the last paragraph of the Terms of Service (paragraph 51) incorporates into the Terms of Service all the NHS (General Medical Services) Regulations 1992 as amended, and specified parts of Part 2 of the NHS (Service Committee and Tribunal) Regulations 1974 as amended.

Certain provisions of the Terms of Service may cause problems. Some of these are listed below and require special attention.

Patients

The doctor's patients are not just those on his list. Read paragraph 4 carefully.

Medical card

The medical card should be sent to the FHSA within 14 days of acceptance (paragraph 6).

Child health and minor surgery (Regulations 27, 28, 32 and 33)

Before applying to undertake these services, it is essential to read these Regulations and Schedule 3, Parts VIII, IX and Schedules 4 and 6 very carefully.

Terminating responsibility for patients (paragraphs 9–11)

Note the case of the patient under treatment, the provisions for maternity services, the termination of child health surveillance when a child is examined outside the practice (Regulation 28(3)(d)) and the need to inform the Authority and the parent in writing (Regulation 28(4)(a) and (b)).

Nature of service to patients (paragraphs 12, 13, 14, 15, 16)

These are the paragraphs under which a doctor is most likely to be found in breach at a service committee. They should be read carefully, in conjunction with paragraph 3. Failure to visit and failure to perform a full examination under paragraph 12 and 13 are the most difficult events to defend. However, patients may, in future, complain about the failure to detect or prevent disease under paragraphs 14 (new registrations), 15 (not seen within 3 years) or 16 (over 75s). The mere fact that the examinations prescribed under 14(2), 15(4) or 16(5) have been carried out will not be an adequate defence if, for any reason, a more extensive examination was indicated. It follows that particular care is needed if any part of this work is delegated to a nurse. Comprehensive and detailed records, made at the time, are the most valuable protection.

Deputizing (paragraph 18–26)

A doctor, not on the obstetric list, may *only* deputize for a doctor on the list in an obstetric emergency as defined in paragraph 19(7). Curiously, this seems to require him to ensure that such an emergency exists, or could exist, before attending. For child health services, it is possible to request the consent of the Authority to employ a deputy *not* on the relevant list. The Authority must be informed of arrangements for the employment of a deputy on a regular basis and of the name of the doctor or doctors responsible for the practice when a doctor proposes to be absent from the practice for more than one week (paragraph 21(2)).

Availability

The rules are contained in paragraphs 29–30. Note that a doctor is free to choose on which 5 days he is to be available but the allocation of hours between the chosen days should be convenient to patients (paragraph 29(2)(b)). In calculating the times at which a doctor is regarded as available, he may include clinics and time spent actually making domiciliary visits (paragraph 29(7)) and 'availability' shall be construed accordingly.

Practice area (paragraph 34)

Note that practice area has the specific meaning assigned in Regulation 2 (Interpretation). It is, therefore, peculiar to the doctor rather than his practice and each partner may have a different practice area. This should be made clear if a joint practice leaflet is prepared (paragraph 47) and Schedule 12.

Certification (paragraph 37)

Schedule 9 to the NHS (General Medical and Pharmaceutical Services) Regulations 1974 contains the list of certificates a doctor must issue to patients *or their representatives* free of charge. Certificates have to be reasonably required and patients have to be attended by, or under the supervision of, the doctor, his partner or his deputy. If the doctor is not medically attending the patient (e.g. if the patient is being attended solely by another practitioner or consultant), there is no obligation to issue a certificate although the doctor may, if he wishes, issue a special statement based on a written report made by the other doctor. The detailed rules for the issue of statements are to be found in departmental guidance, *Medical evidence for Social Security and Statutory Sick Pay purposes*. However, the most important aspect of certification is to ensure that every statement or certificate issued is absolutely and literally truthful.

Fees

Paragraph 38 contains the list of fees a doctor is entitled to demand and accept from a patient for whose treatment he is responsible. Note that a doctor can demand fees from a patient as long as it is not for 'treatment' but 'treatment' means 'medical attendance and treatment' (Regulation 2). This raises the untested but intriguing question of whether a doctor may charge patients for non-attendance at missed appointments.

Prescribing

Paragraph 43 makes it clear that a doctor can only issue an NHS prescription to a patient to whom he, the doctor, is providing treatment under his terms of service. Since treatment means medical attendance and treatment (Regulation 2), the doctor cannot prescribe for a patient who is being medically attended solely by someone else (other than the doctor's partner or deputy acting under paragraph 19(2)). Prescriptions must be signed in ink by the doctor *after* the particulars have been inserted on the form. Never sign blank prescription forms. Never prescribe a drug for whose choice, dose and supervision you are not prepared to take personal responsibility. Drugs in Schedule 10 may not be prescribed and those in Schedule 11 only for the purposes specified.

Practice leaflets

Schedule 12 details the information which must be included (paragraph 47). The doctor must review the leaflet annually and amend it as necessary to maintain accuracy. It is worth noting that a leaflet does not have to be printed. A typewritten leaflet giving the prescribed information complies with the rules as long as a (photo)copy is sent to the FHSA and is available to each patient on the list. As long as the statutory leaflet is available, other practice literature – practice cards, timetables, handbooks etc – need not contain all the prescribed information.

Annual reports

Schedule 13 details the information which must be included (paragraph 50).

Whilst the Regulations are not an easy read, it is important that every GP is aware of their content, and in particular of the sections dealing with Terms of Service, the provision of services and the rights of access to those services by patients. Every practice should have a set of Regulations for reference purposes, and expert help and advice on matters of interpretation can be obtained from Local Medical Committee secretaries or from the BMA regional offices.

4 Service Committee and Tribunal Regulations

John Oldroyd

THE Statutory instrument 644, NHS (Service Committee and Tribunal) Regulations 1992 is the Apocrypha of the NHS. A dictionary definition of apocrypha is 'hidden or secret things'.

This definition indicates the attitude most GPs should have to the minutiae of this statutory instrument. They should be aware of its existence but when its provisions threaten to become part of their lives they should seek guidance from those whose job it is to be familiar with the detail. Those who have familiarity are the medical secretaries of the defence bodies, Local Medical Committee (LMC) secretaries and perhaps colleagues who may have served as LMC nominees on the service committees of the Family Health Services Authority (FHSA).

This chapter gives an outline of the regulations: it does not substitute for the depth of advice an individual will require if he becomes involved in a complaint to the FHSA against him.

The provision of regulations

These detail the basis for admission of complaints made against an NHS contractor be he doctor, dentist, chemist or optician to an FHSA and the procedure for dealing with such complaints.

In addition the regulations describe procedures for investigation of:

1 excessive prescribing by a doctor;
2 National Insurance certification;
3 clinical record keeping;
4 whether a substance prescribed by a doctor was a drug the NHS is bound to provide;
5 the powers of Local Representative Committees (i.e. the LMC for doctors) to investigate matters brought to their attention by a doctor 'involving any question of the efficiency of the general medical services'.

The remainder of this chapter deals only with complaints in so far as they affect doctors but with regard to 1, 2 and 3 above, advice should always be taken if faced with such an investigation before making any response.

Complaints

The Regulations deal with two sources of complaint as far as they relate to doctors:

1 regarding care of patients in relation to GP's terms of service;
2 regarding administration in relation to the terms of service.

Administration

Investigations by a service committee (*vide infra*) have been possible under this heading for many years, but cases brought were few and far between. However, the introduction of the 1990 contract with its increased obligations, e.g. provision of practice leaflets, annual reports, three yearly health checks, offers of annual consultations to the over 75s etc, may occasion use of this provision by FHSAs themselves much more frequently in the future. With certain important variations the mechanisms are similar to those described below.

Service to patients

For a formal investigation to proceed the complaint should relate to an allegation of a prima facie breach in the terms of service for doctors contained in the schedule to the main NHS regulations. However, issued with the consolidated Service Committee and Tribunal Regulations by the Department of Health in 1990 are extensive Notes of Guidance. At the time of writing, the Notes of Guidance to the 1992 Consolidated Regulations have not been published. One section of these notes stresses the use of informal procedures to try and resolve matters before 'entering a formal complaint'.

Informal procedure

FHSAs are not constrained to using informal means of resolving matters that only strictly fall outside alleged breaches in terms of service.

Minor allegations of breach of terms of service may also be considered. Use of the informal procedure does not preclude a formal investigation if matters are not resolved.

Whilst the Notes of Guidance suggest a mechanism for informal procedures by use of a lay conciliator with medical advice, not all FHSAs have instituted such a mechanism. Many and various are the informal procedures currently in use. However, GPs should try to use the informal process in their own locality if offered, as experience shows a large number of complaints are resolved by these mechanisms.

Formal procedures

Formal procedures are laid down precisely in the regulations. Like all regulations they are subject to amendment. The last major amendment was in 1992 after consultation and consolidated regulations incorporating all current amendments were issued for implementation from 1 April 1992.

The Medical Service Committee

Each FHSA is required to set up a subcommittee known as the Medical Service Committee (MSC), to investigate complaints against doctors. It is comprised of three lay people, three GPs nominated by the LMC and a lay chairman appointed by the FHSA.

The chairman's role is an important one in the initial investigation of complaints. When a complaint is received by the FHSA and it is not suitable for, or fails to be resolved by, the informal procedure the chairman must decide if the allegations suggest a prima facie breach of the terms of service. If so, is the complaint made by a person properly entitled to complain in terms of the regulations (usually the patient involved or a person acting with the authority of the patient when the patient is alive, or by *anyone* when the patient is dead), and is it made within the statutory time limit (13 weeks from the incident)?

The complaint having been so adjudged, the GP (the practitioner) is informed by letter of the complaint. Usually the letter of complaint is also sent as complaints are required to be in writing when presented to the doctor and it will be pointed out which paragraph of the terms of service are deemed to have been alleged to have been breached. (There are special rules for oral complaints made to the FHSA.) The doctor is invited within a period of 30 days, to submit his comments (a longer period may be allowed on application) and advised to seek guidance from his LMC or defence body.

The most important thing to do next is to take advice before replying to the FHSA. The content of the response letter is crucial to the whole subsequent development of the complaint.

Whether the adviser is from the LMC or the defence body there are two ways of advising. The first would be for the doctor to submit all the correspondence to the adviser together with his thought-out reply for amendment or approval. The second would be at a meeting between doctor and adviser to go through the details of the complaint with a view to obtaining advice on the drafting of a suitable reply. In either case the adviser will need to see any supporting evidence, the most important of which is the patient's notes. Depending on the circumstances the adviser may require statements from staff, deputies, ambulance services or anyone else involved. Hospital letters and post mortem reports may also be of value.

Essentially the adviser will be:

1 looking to present a considered narrative of the events from the doctor's point of view;
2 looking at the legal correctness of the complaint in terms of the regulations, e.g.

   (a) Was the complaint laid in terms of the regulations by a person entitled to complain or with such a person's authority?
   (b) Was the complaint made in the time limits specified in the regulations? If not, should one be prepared to give consent to investigations of part or the whole of a complaint outside those limits? If consent is not given what should the doctor's attitude be to the FHSA accepting a complainant's reason for delay and then seeking the Secretary of State's authority to proceed with the investigation?

   In fact most experienced advisers are aware of cases when the Secretary of State has not given such authority when the respondent doctor has refused consent. However, only the experience of an adviser can determine whether such 'tactics' are sensible or justified in the long-term interests of the doctor.

3 prognosticating on how the complaint will proceed: seeing and reading the case. This will entail: looking at the complaint from the point of view of a third party; seeing where the Service Committee

will see areas of difficulty/weakness and need for correlation. The adviser will plan the assembly of the supporting evidence that may require presentation at the time of the initial response or to be introduced later.

What is not needed in this initial response is an ill-judged reflex riposte about the complainant's ingratitude, difficult personality, morals, hygiene and mental ineptitude. Slanging matches are not to be entered into no matter how hurt the recipient of the complaint may feel about the allegations. Equally, gaps in the narrative which beg further questions can lead to further difficulties as matters proceed.

A good adviser will appreciate the legal nuances. They should be an expert at both teasing out parts of the sequence of events that may seem unimportant to an interested party, and judging the effect of a draft response on the Service Committee chairman, or if matters go to a hearing, on the members.

Once a response has been prepared, then it is returned to the FHSA. This will be sent on to the complainant who is invited to respond to it. A number of complainants having received a 'reasoned' reply, which may or may not be conciliatory, withdraw the complaint (or do not bother to pursue it further) at this stage.

Although the FHSA has the power the continue an investigation that is not pursued by the complainant this rarely happens. However, in the bulk of cases the complainant does reply. The respondent doctor may or may not be invited to give comments on this reply, but in reality at this stage the Service Committee chairman decides either that the correspondence completely answers the allegations of a breach in the Terms of Service or it does not. If it does answer the allegation then correspondence is presented to a meeting of the Service Committee with a view that the complaint does not merit further examination and can therefore be dismissed. The Service Committee can agree – and so dismissal is recommended to the FHSA – or disagree. In cases of disagreement, or where the chairman himself decide further consideration is necessary, the parties are informed that a hearing is to be arranged.

The hearing

The procedures in the preparation for a hearing and at the hearing itself are laid down in Schedule 4 of the Regulations and the account that follows is only a brief outline, but covers all the essential points.

Preliminary

The FHSA is required to:

1 give notice to both parties that there will be a hearing;
2 indicate what Terms of Service are alleged to have been breached;
3 inform the parties of the names of the members of the Service Committee;
4 request from the parties any documentary evidence they wish to submit within 14 days which will be furnished to the other party and the names of witnesses to be called;
5 notify the members of the Service Committee and supply them with correspondence.

Where more than one doctor is involved, the complaint is usually addressed to the doctor on whose list the patient is registered. However, where the complaint is solely related to the actions of a deputy then there are two differing situations depending on whether the doctor deputizing is: (a) a doctor also in contract for the FHSA, i.e. on the list; or (b) a doctor not in contract (e.g. a trainee, locum or other deputy).

Where a doctor in contract is involved the complaint may also be directed against him and he will have been involved in the early correspondence. If the Service Committee considers there has been no failing on the part of the patient's registered doctor they will dispense with any hearing involving his part and recommend dismissal. The hearing will be with the deputy respondent.

Where a deputizing doctor is not in contract then the patient's registered doctor is considered responsible for the actions of such a deputy and it will be against the responsible doctor that the complaint is directed. The other doctor may be brought to a hearing as a witness, but he has the important right of applying within 30 days of the statement of a hearing being called, to become a party to the investigation.

This in effect means that such a deputy can attend the whole of a hearing and consequently hear precisely the evidence of the complaint and contribute to and receive documentary evidence. No sanctions, as he has no contract, can be brought against him. However, it should be stressed that the same right does not apply to non-medically qualified persons. Thus complaints against practice staff are made against the registered doctor who is responsible for their actions and practice receptionists, managerial and nursing staff can only be introduced as witnesses at hearings.

From the respondent's point of view it will now be obvious that with only 30 days notice, and 14 days to present the documentary evidence and names of witnesses, time is short. It is important to anticipate what will be required and consult in advance with the adviser.

Since April 1990, complainant and respondent, have been allowed the right to be represented not only by a friend but also by an official – provided that he is not legally qualified from an organization to which they belong. This means that the complainant may have a Community Health Council secretary or member present the case; and the doctor a representative of the LMC (usually the secretary or his assistant) or a secretary from his defence body. Prior to 1990 such individuals could attend the hearing only as advisers. They were not allowed to address the Service Committee directly, but they could advise the party in whispers. Such a role is still allowed.

Although there are attractions to having a representative act as one's advocate, there are drawbacks. Shielding a doctor from the Service Committee at a hearing can diminish the important impact of a doctor's sincerity. The role of the LMC secretary of defence body secretary as representative/adviser should be discussed and decided upon before the hearing and all the implications considered.

At the hearing itself, whilst an outline for procedure is given in the schedule, the actual conduct is at the discretion of the chairman.

To be quorate at a hearing there have to be at least two lay and two professional members as well as the lay chairman. All must declare they have no interest. In this context there is provision for the investigation/hearing to be passed to an FHSA other than the one with whom the doctor has his contract, and this clearly applies when the FHSA is itself the complainant or when the doctor (or complainant) is well known to the service committee (e.g. a member of the committee).

The procedure usually followed is for the complainant or his representative to present his case, remembering that the committee have read the correspondence and written evidence. He is then questioned by the other party and then by the committee. Witnesses are introduced, their evidence elicited by questioning by the complainant; followed by questioning by the respondent and the committee. When this is completed, the situation is reversed. The respondent or his representative presents the response. Questions and witnesses follow the same pattern.

Both parties are then given an opportunity to sum up. They are then informed by the chairman that they will hear the outcome of proceedings after the subcommittee (i.e. Service Committee) report has been considered by the full FHSA at a subsequent meeting. Both parties then withdraw.

The Service Committee then go on to determine whether the respondent doctor was in breach or not. If they feel he was not then this ends their deliberations. The decision is taken on a majority vote of members. In the event of a tie the chairman has the deciding vote. In matters involving clinical management and skills the lay members should be advised by professional members.

If a breach is found then the Service Committee makes recommendations to the FHSA. These recommendations relate to the powers of the FHSA to take action. They may take into account any previous findings of breach by the same respondent in the past 6 years. Their recommendations may include that:

1 the practitioner be warned to comply more closely with his Terms of Service in future;
2 there be a withholding from remuneration. Where this is below £500 the FHSA can determine the amount themselves. Where it is over £500 the FHSA recommends to the Secretary of State such a withholding;
3 where, after consultation with the LMC, the number of patients on the doctor's list is considered to be excessive and he is unable to give them all adequate treatment, a limit on the numbers should be applied. (This is rarely used);
4 where the continued inclusion of the name of the doctor is prejudicial to the efficiency of the NHS there be reference to a Tribunal.

Service Committees are not empowered to make recommendations concerning practice organization or monitoring of a doctor's performance by their FHSA medical advisers, and they must confine their recommendations to those listed above.

The report of the Service Committee is prepared and presented to the FHSA. Usually it is adopted without modification, but FHSAs have the power to both vary findings and recommendations.

After the FHSA determination, copies of the report are sent to both parties, notifying them of their right of appeal to the Secretary of State.

Privacy

Investigations are meant to be private and confidential. Over and above their role as the respondent's adviser the LMC secretary or representative of the LMC may attend the hearing as an observer; and members of either House of Parliament are entitled to a copy of the report as a response to a request from either party.

The FHSA can, when an appeal period is over, release details to the press of Service Committee cases suitably anonymized so the parties cannot be identified.

Appeals to the Secretary of State

Notice of appeal must be given within 30 days and must be based on reasons more cogent than that the adverse findings or recommendations were unpalatable. Appeals by the respondent may be against the finding of breach or the severity of recommendation.

From 1 April 1992 the Secretary of State has devolved his appeal function to Yorkshire Regional Health Authority who have set up an FHS Appeals Unit at Harrogate.

Appeal hearings

These are held before three appointees of the Appeals Unit, at least one of whom will be from a panel nominated by a body recognized as representative of NHS GPs (i.e. the General Medical Services Committee of the BMA). In essence this is a rehearing of the Service Committee but the parties are entitled to legal representation. There is a provision for costs to be allowable if so determined by the appeal body. The findings are incorporated in a report. The decision on this report is final.

Clearly any doctor contemplating an appeal should consult his defence body for advice and the necessary legal support.

Medical Advisory Committee (MAC)

The Regulations require the Secretary of State to set up this body to advise him on his duties in regard to the withholding of monies 'and in any other case'. The MAC is chaired by a doctor 'who has been engaged in the provision of services under the Act for not less than 10 years', and has been selected after consultation with the GMSC.

This function of the Secretary of State has been developed to Regional Health Authorities, with a central Appeals Unit based at Yorkshire RHA acting on behalf of all regions. The profession's role on this new MAC has not changed.

The MAC have the role of equating at a national level, the severity of recommendations by the various local bodies. Where a MAC increases the level of withholding recommended by an FHSA there are provisions for representation by the respondent.

The tribunal

This is the body which can determine whether or not a doctor should be allowed to continue as an NHS GP. The chairman is an office holder 'during the pleasure of the Lord Chancellor'. Obviously a doctor facing such a body should take legal advice if he has not already done so.

The General Medical Council

Reference by FHSAs to the General Medical Council (GMC), where breaches are disclosed, are not encouraged by the Secretary of State. In the current Notes of Guidance this advice is being reviewed in the light of the recent introduction of the FHSA's own autonomy in determining cases with withholdings up to £500. Rather does the Secretary of State take on himself the role of reporting cases where thought appropriate to the GMC. In this he is advised by the MAC and this body in turn has been advised by the GMC. No specific indication that a given case will or will not be referred can be given but the cases listed below and as stated in the Notes of Guidance are likely to be referred.

1 Certain cases involving neglect or disregard of professional responsibilities to patients.
2 Directions by the NHS Tribunal that a doctor's name should be removed from the Medical List.
3 Cases of irregular certification under National Insurance rules.

4 Cases of irregular charging of fees to patients.

5 Cases concerning fraud or improper claim to fees.

6 Cases where there may have been canvassing or gaining of patients by unethical means.

FHSA's like any other body have a right and, in certain circumstances, a duty to refer cases of professional misconduct that come to their attention – some such cases may be outside the Services Committee and Tribunal Regulations.

Further reading

Department of Health *Family Practitioner Services complaints procedure, Notes of Guidance to the FPS complaints procedure.*

Statutory Instrument (1992) No. 664 *The NHS. (Service Committees and Tribunal) Regulations 1992.*

The Medical Protection Society *General practice complaints procedure.*

The Medical Defence Union *Complaints to FPCs.*

Owen C (1990) Formal complaints against general practitioners: A study of 1000 cases. *British Journal of General Practice*, 4; 113–115.

5   Doctors and Dispensing

Gareth Emrys-Jones

Who may dispense medication?

THE Medicines Act 1968 empowers all doctors to dispense medication, provided that the terms of the Act, covering such issues as the safe custody of medicines, record keeping, labelling and standards of containers are complied with. The Medicines Act is comprehensive and applies to all doctors. Other Acts that are applicable to all doctors include the Medicines (Labelling) Regulations 1976–1985, Misuse of Drugs Regulations 1985 (England and Wales), the Medicines (Child Safety) Regulations 1975–1976, the National Health Service Charges for Drugs and Appliances Regulations 1980 and Part 1 of the Consumer Protection Act 1987.

The National Health Service (Pharmaceutical Services) Regulations 1992, define the circumstances when a practitioner **must** provide pharmaceutical services to his patients, and when a practitioner **may** provide such services, and receive payment for doing so.

Provision of pharmaceutical services by doctors

Regulation 19 (NHS Pharmaceutical Regulations 1992) states that: '*A doctor (a) shall provide to a patient any appliance or drug, not being a Scheduled drug, where such provision is needed for the immediate treatment of that patient before a provision can otherwise be obtained; and (b) may provide to a patient any appliance or drug not being a Scheduled drug, which he personally administers, or applies to that patient.*'

Sub-paragraph (a) is a requirement of all practitioners; and sub-paragraph (b) enables all doctors to claim payment under Paragraph 44.5 of the Statement of Fees and Allowances (SFA) for personally administered items.

Box 5.1:
1 The Medicines Act enables *all* doctors to dispense.
2 The NHS Acts define when a practitioner *must* dispense, and under what circumstances a practitioner *may* claim payment for dispensing.

In fulfilling the requirement of sub-paragraph (a) practitioners must be mindful of the legislation covering controlled drugs, labelling requirements and the product liability law.

Controlled drugs

The relevant Regulations concerning controlled drugs are the Misuse of Drugs Act 1971, Dangerous Drugs The Misuse of Drugs Regulations 1985 and subsequent amendments.

Box 5.2:
For controlled drugs there are special rules for:
1 who can possess and supply;
2 record keeping;
3 storage;
4 prescription writing.

Possession and supply

The Misuse of Drugs Regulations authorizes practitioners to both possess and supply controlled drugs. These are defined in Schedules 1 to 5 of the same regulations. Medicinal products are in the main included in Schedule 2 (opiates and amphetamines), Schedule 3 (appetite suppressants) and Schedule 4 (benzodiazepines.)

Records

Regulation 19 of the Misuse of Drugs Regulations requires any person authorized to possess or supply a controlled drug to maintain a register in an approved form of the quantity of all controlled drugs obtained and supplied, including any administered personally. All entries are to be made in chronological order. A separate part of the register is to be maintained for each class of drugs mentioned in the schedules, and for each individual drug.

Regulation 20 of the Misuse of Drugs Regulations specifies the requirements for maintaining the register. These include:

1 the entry must be made on the day of the transaction, or on the following day;
2 the entry must be made in ink or otherwise so as to be indelible;
3 there must be no cancellations, obliterations or alterations. If a correction has to be made it may only be done by way of a marginal note or a footnote which must be dated;
4 a register must be kept at each place to which it relates. This means that a practitioner who carries a controlled drug to personally administer to a patient must carry and maintain a register;
5 a register must be kept for a minimum of 2 years after the date of the last entry.

Storage

All controlled drugs must be kept in a locked receptacle that can only be opened by the doctor or with his authority (Misuse of Drugs (Safe Custody) Regulations). It has been held in the High Court that a locked car is not an adequate receptacle for the storage of controlled drugs.

Prescribing controlled drugs

A prescription for a controlled drug must:

1 be written in ink, or otherwise so as to be indelible, and must be signed and dated by the person issuing it with his usual signature;
2 be written by the person issuing it in his own handwriting;
3 specify the name and address of the person for whom it is intended;
4 specify the strength of the preparation, the dose to be taken and the quantity of the preparation in both words and figures.

A prescription for phenobarbitone or a compound containing phenobarbitone, and no other controlled drug, need not comply with the handwriting regulation.

Containers

Any doctor providing pharmaceutical services to patients shall supply any medication in a suitable container (NHS Pharmaceutical Regulations, Schedule 2, Part III. Terms of Service for Doctors Para 11(b)).

Suitable containers

These are defined in Part IV of the Drug Tariff in the following terms: '*Capsules, tablets, pills, pulvules etc shall be supplied in airtight containers of glass, aluminium or rigid plastic; card containers may be used only for foil/strip packed tablets etc. For ointments, creams, pastes, card containers shall not be used. Eye, ear and nasal drops shall be supplied in dropper bottles or with a separate dropper where appropriate*'.

As a safety measure all containers used for the supply of medication should be reclosable and child-resistant, unless the patient is elderly or handicapped and would have difficulty in opening a child-resistant container.

A 5 ml plastic measuring spoon shall be supplied with every oral liquid medicine, unless a patient already has a spoon or the manufacturer's pack contains one.

Labelling

The Medicines (Labelling) Regulations 1976–85 require that any medication dispensed, whether by a doctor, or on the instructions of a doctor, must be labelled. Such a label must include:

1 the name of the person to whom the medicine is to be given;
2 the name and address of the supplier. (In the case of a doctor dispensing the medication the name and address of that doctor or partnership);
3 the date the prescription was dispensed;
4 the words 'keep out of reach of children'.

There is no legal requirement, but it is deemed to be good practice, to include the name of the preparation, instructions for use and any appropriate warnings.

Product liability

Part 1 of the Consumer Protection Act 1987 removes the need for a person who suffers damage as a result of taking a drug to prove negligence. It is now only necessary to prove that the product was defective and that any damage caused was a result of such a defect.

The liability falls on the manufacturer or importer. Where neither of these is identifiable liability will rest with the supplier unless he can identify a person higher up the distribution chain, for example a wholesaler.

It is therefore imperative that doctors maintain a record of each drug supplied to every patient. This should be kept in the patient's record. Record should also be kept of all invoices so as to identify the source of every drug. These records should be kept for at least 11 years.

Prescription forms

A prescription form is defined in NHS (General Medical Services) Regulations 1992, Schedule 2 paragraph 1 as: *'a form provided by a health Authority, an FHSA or, where the doctor is on the medical list of more than one FHSA, by the FHSA which is responsible for the supply of that form, and issued by a doctor to enable a person to obtain pharmaceutical services.'*

A doctor is required to order any drugs, chemical agents or appliances which are needed for the treatment of any patient to whom he is providing treatment under the Terms of Service by issuing to that patient a prescription form. If the doctor is empowered, under Regulation 20 of the NHS (Pharmaceutical Services) Regulations 1992, to provide dispensing services for that patient, the order for the supply of a drug shall be made on a prescription form but there is no requirement to issue the form to the patient.

Box 5.3:
An order for medication to be supplied to a patient receiving NHS treatment must be made on a prescription form (FP10).

Under the provision of Regulation 20(8) NHS (Pharmaceutical Services) Regulations 1992, a doctor may issue, with the patient's consent a prescription form to enable the patient who is on his doctor's dispensing list to obtain a supply of medication from elsewhere.

A prescription form issued to a patient is thus an order to supply the relevant medication to that patient. A prescription form for a dispensing patient is a record of supply of the medication and becomes, on presentation to the Prescription Pricing Authority, a request for payment.

A doctor is required to sign each prescription form in ink with his initials or forenames and surname in his own handwriting and not by means of a stamp. Each form is only to be signed after the particulars on the form have been inserted.

Box 5.4:
A prescription form must be signed by a doctor only after the particulars have been filled in.

A prescription shall not refer to any previous prescription and a separate prescription form shall be issued for each patient unless the doctor is prescribing in bulk for a school or institution under paragraph 45 Schedule 2 (Terms of Service for doctors) NHS Regulations 1992.

A doctor is prohibited from:

1 ordering on a prescription form a preparation included in Schedule 10 (NHS (General Medical Services) Regulations 1992 (the 'Black List')); or

2 supplying under pharmaceutical services a patient on his dispensing list with a preparation included in Schedule 10. A doctor may however supply such a preparation to a patient on his dispensing list, otherwise than under pharmaceutical services, and may demand or accept a fee from the patient in respect of such a supply.

Prescription charges

A doctor who supplies drugs or appliances to a patient, except where supplied under the immediate treatment provision (Regulation 19 NHS Pharmaceutical Services Regulations 1992), is obliged to make and recover a charge for each item. The Regulations covering prescription charges are the National Health Service (Charges for Drugs and Appliances) Regulations 1980. These Regulations cover the recovery of charges by chemists and dispensing doctors and hospital out-patient departments. It includes sections on exemptions, prepayment and any repayment, by an Authority, to a patient.

Paragraph 4 requires a doctor who has dispensed medication, to make and recover a charge, the level of which is determined periodically by the Government, from the patient unless the patient, or a person acting on behalf of the patient, declares that he is entitled to exemption from the charge.

If the patient is not exempt the doctor is under no obligation to supply any medication unless he is first paid the appropriate charge.

The doctor who recovers a charge in these circumstances, if so requested by a patient, is obliged to issue a receipt on a form provided by the FHSA to enable the patient to obtain reimbursement, if so entitled from the FHSA.

A doctor is required to forward each month, to the FHSA, any monies so collected.

Provision of pharmaceutical services by doctors

The regulations governing the provision of pharmaceutical services to patients by doctors are complex.

The relevant regulations are included in the National Health Service (Pharmaceutical Services) Regulations 1992. The relevant paragraphs applying to doctors and pharmacists in rural areas are 9 to 14 and 19 to 21. There are also departmental guidelines (HSG(92)13 Pharmaceutical Services).

Any doctor either wishing to commence dispensing or being involved in an application by a pharmacist to start dispensing in a rural area should consult the above guidelines and regulations.

Arrangements for the provision of pharmaceutical services by doctors

Prior to 1 April 1983 any doctor, if requested to do so by a patient living in a rural area, could provide pharmaceutical services for that patient.

Any doctor who was supplying drugs or appliances to patients prior to 1 April 1983, or who is in a practice where a partner or a former principal in the practice was supplying drugs or appliances to patients prior to 1 April 1983, may continue to do so.

He may accept on to his dispensing list any patient who is resident in a controlled locality, at a distance of more than 1 mile as the crow flies from any pharmacy and at least one of the following conditions apply to that patient:

1 that he has not previously been included on a doctor's list;
2 he has changed his address from that last notified to a committee; or
3 he has not changed address but immediately before acceptance by a doctor he was being provided with pharmaceutical services by a doctor.

Alternatively if there is in effect an outline consent granted persuant to the regulations, a doctor may accept any patient living in a controlled locality at a distance of more than 1 mile as the crow flies from any pharmacy, for the provision of pharmaceutical services.

The application for pharmaceutical services has to be made by the patient himself (if over 16 years of age) and has to be in writing.

Unless the doctor has been granted outline consent the application should be made at the same time as the application to join the doctor's list for the provision of general medical services in order to comply with the three conditions above.

Box 5.6:
Unless outline consent to dispense has been granted, an application by a patient to be included on a doctor's dispensing list must be made at the time of registration.

Determination of a controlled locality

Regulation 9(1), National Health Service (Pharmaceutical Regulations) 1992, specifies that where an area had been determined prior to 17 September 1990, either by a Family Practitioner Committee, as then was, or by the Rural Dispensing Committee under regulation 30F as was then in force, to be rural in character that area shall be a controlled locality.

The rurality of an area may be reviewed at any time by an FHSA, and must be reviewed on an application by either a Local Pharmaceutical or Local Medical Committee.

Outline consent to dispense

A doctor who wishes to provide pharmaceutical services under these regulations may at any time apply to the FHSA for consent to do so.

An FHSA is obliged to **refuse** any application, if the granting of the application would prejudice the proper provision of general medical or pharmaceutical services in any area. It shall also **refuse** any application that relates to an area that is not a controlled locality or is within 1 mile of any pharmacy. Subject to the above the FHSA is obliged to **grant** any application.

An FHSA is empowered to impose conditions to mitigate any adverse effects the granting of the application may have on any doctor or pharmacist.

The FHSA is not allowed to consider any application where there has been a decision reached within the 5 years immediately preceding the application, unless there has been a substantial change of circumstances affecting the controlled locality.

Appeals against an FHSA decision

General

Appeals against an FHSA decision are to the Regional Health Authority (RHA). The RHAs have decided that all appeals shall be heard by Yorkshire RHA who, to that end, have established an Appeals Unit. All action resulting from an appeal will be taken by the Appeals Unit.

A decision on an appeal, made by the Appeals Unit is not reviewable by the RHA from whose region the appeal arose.

All appeals should be sent directly to the Yorkshire RHA FHS Appeals Unit at: FHS Appeal Unit, Yorkshire Health, Rooms 24–26 Fourth Floor, Windsor House, Cornwall Road, Harrogate HG1 2PW.

Appeals relating to the rurality of an area

Appeals relating to the rurality of an area can only be made by the Local Medical Committee or the Local Pharmaceutical Committee.

Any appeal must be made within 1 month from the date when the decision was sent to the Local Representative Committee.

Appeals can only be made against an FHSA's decision:

1 that the area is or is not rural;
2 that it refuses to consider the rurality of the area on the grounds that it is not satisfied that there has been a substantial change in circumstance in any part of the area since the question was last determined. (An FHSA is not allowed consider the rurality of an area within 5 years of a decision on the rurality being reached, unless there has been a substantial change in circumstances in that area);
3 that measures are, or are not, required to reduce any adverse consequences of a decision.

Appeals relating to grant of outline or preliminary consent

Where an FHSA has granted or refused an application for outline consent by a doctor, or preliminary consent by a pharmacist, the applicant or any person who is on either the medical or pharmaceutical list of the FHSA and who was sent copies of the application and who has submitted written evidence concerning the application to the FHSA, may appeal in writing within 1 month from the date on which notice of the decision was sent to the appellant.

Notice of an appeal shall be sent to any person who was notified of the application and who submitted written evidence to the FHSA.

It is for this reason that it is important to ensure that any practitioner, and any Local Medical Committee that receives notice of an application, always submit some written comment on the initial application or else they will be excluded from any appeal consideration.

6 Dealing with Death

John Burton

FOR many medical students their undergraduate education on dealing with death will have emphasized the explanation of death to relatives and support for them during their bereavement. However, in order to deal confidently with death, doctors must have a clear understanding of the law, particularly relating to certification. In dealing with deaths, doctors have two distinct functions:

1 confirming that life is extinct;
2 issuing a certificate for the registrar in directing the cause of death, and/or informing the coroner.

Many countries have a system where only some types of death are investigated. In England and Wales however a system has evolved that uses the 'fail safe' principle. Every death has to be investigated by the coroner at an inquest held in public *unless* it can be proved that the death was due to natural causes. The information needed to show that an inquest is not required comes from two sources. If the deceased person was attended by a registered medical practitioner in the course of the illness that caused the death, that practitioner must issue a certificate of the cause of death. This is scrutinized by the registrar of deaths, who will only register the death, if satisfied that the case does not have to be referred to the coroner, or if not refer the matter to the coroner. The second source of information comes from the power of the coroner to order a post mortem examination of the body in cases of a sudden death where the cause is unknown (Section 19, Coroners Act 1988). If this shows that an inquest is not necessary, the coroner informs the registrar of deaths and the death can be registered. Thus, every death that is not shown to be due to a natural cause must be the subject of a coroner's inquest. The fact that a death is referred to the coroner does not imply that there is a suspicion of foul play. It merely indicates that there is not the proof required to show that the death is due to a known, natural cause.

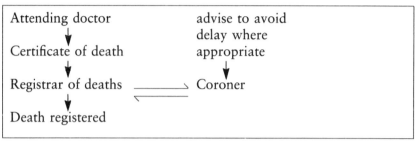

Figure 6.1:

Death certificate

The majority of deaths in England are expected and due to a natural cause. Where a patient has been attended by a registered medical practitioner in the last illness (the illness that caused the death) that practitioner is obliged, under Section 22 of the Births and Deaths Registration Act 1953, to complete a certificate in the prescribed form, stating the cause of death to the best of his knowledge and to deliver

CAUSE OF DEATH	
The condition thought to be the 'Underlying Cause of Death' should appear in the lowest completed line of Part I.	These particulars not to be entered in death register
	Approximate interval between onset and death
	....
I(a) Disease or condition .... directly leading to death	
(b) Other disease or condition, ... if any, leading to I(a)	....
(c) Other disease or condition, ... if any, leading to I(b)	....
II Other significant conditions CONTRIBUTING TO THE DEATH but not related to the disease or condition causing it.	....

Figure 6.2: Extract from death certificate

that certificate to the registrar of deaths. The doctor is not obliged to see the body, in order to certify the death, but it is exceptional not to do so. (For cremations forms, *see* page 66). The obligation on the attending doctor to certify is absolute, even when the death is known to be an unnatural one. (*see* page 63, 64 and 65 regarding discussion with the coroner.)

The registrar general provides the certificates in books. The cover has full instructions for completing the forms printed on it; and it is essential that all doctors who are likely to have to certify death read this information before they issue a certificate. The cause of death is given in accordance with the international classification and it performs two functions:

1 it informs the registrar of deaths whether the death was natural or unnatural;
2 it informs the statisticians of the underlying cause of death.

If the cause of death was natural, then the final line should disclose this, e.g. 1a Myocardial infarction due to 1b Coronary atheroma. Abbreviations should not be used and, if the terms used could apply to a number of causes of death, it must be explained by the line underneath. Thus hepatic failure could be due to infiltration by a malignant growth or to paracetamol poisoning; septicaemia could be from a natural infection or following an injury. It is sometimes difficult to find an explanation, e.g. where a person has died from progressive deterioration of all organs due to old age. Multi-organ failure, due to generalized atherosclerosis, may be a compromise.

Secondary cause of death

Part II of the death certificate provides for other contributing conditions to be recorded. It is a part of the cause of death and will be referred to the coroner if it is not manifestly natural. It may be used, for example, where the cause of death was due to the combined effects of a myocardial infarction and chronic obstructive airways disease.

Avoiding delay

There are two problems with the current certificate that the form tries to overcome.

1 If the death is obviously unnatural, there will be a delay while the certificate is delivered to the registrar of deaths and the matter referred to the coroner. The family may be anticipating an early funeral ceremony, and to avoid any problems this may cause, a list of cases that will have to be referred to the coroner is printed on the reverse of the certificate, with a box to mark. If the death has to be referred to the coroner, any delay can be avoided by the doctor informing the coroner's office directly. This can also provide an opportunity to discuss the case.
2 The originating cause of death may be some industrial disease process. There is also a box on the certificate to direct the attention of the certifying doctor to this possibility.

The registrar of deaths

The registrar of deaths is an official who has been trained and instructed by the Office of Population Censuses and Surveys. They are not medically trained or qualified. The instructions given to them are quite specific and are controlled by comprehensive regulations (The Registration of Births and Deaths Regulations 1987). The registrar acts from the information provided by the certificate of death and from information given by the informant, who has attended to register the death. Hence, the wording of the certificate has to be understandable and unambiguous to a layman. The registrar will only register a cause of death that is manifestly due to natural causes and where the patient was attended in the last illness by a registered medical practitioner. Regulation 41 of The Registration of Births and Deaths Regulations 1987 requires that the registrar inform the coroner in any of the following situations:

1 where the deceased was not attended during his last illness by a registered medical practitioner; or
2 where the registrar:

   (a) has been unable to obtain a duly completed certificate of cause of death, or
   (b) has received a certificate which it appears to him, from the particulars contained in the certificate or otherwise, that the deceased was not seen by the certifying medical practitioner either after death or within 14 days before death; or

3 where the cause of death appears to be unknown; or
4 where the registrar has reason to believe the death was unnatural or been caused by violence or neglect or by abortion or to have been attended by suspicious circumstances; or
5 where the death appears to have occurred during an operation or before recovery from the effect of an anaesthetic; or
6 where the death appears to the registrar from the contents of any medical certificate of cause of death to have been due to industrial disease or industrial poisoning.

The registrar will accept chronic alcoholism, cirrhosis of the liver and the medical complications of tobacco smoking as natural causes of death that do not need to be referred to the coroner.

When the death is registered, the registrar of deaths will also give a certificate to permit disposal of the body. Where the body is to be cremated or moved out of England or Wales, additional certificates will be required (*see* page 66 and 67).

Specific problems

One of the most common difficulties is where the deceased has not been seen by the doctor who confirms the death within 14 days prior to the death. This situation may arise where a patient has been treated in hospital and then sent home, or where a patient has attended a practice regularly during his last illness, but was seen by a partner who is on holiday at the time of the death. Discussion with the coroner may allow the coroner to issue Pink Form A to the registrar of deaths and have the death registered from the doctor's certificate.

It must be appreciated that Part (b) of Regulation 41 of the Registration of Births and Deaths Regulation is subordinate to Part (a) (*see* above), i.e. the doctor certifying must have attended during the last illness. If a doctor is treating a patient for an illness that is known to have been the cause of death, there may be some special reason why the doctor has not seen the patient during the 2 weeks preceding death, for example, attendance at hospital or by a partner. The certificate is valid if the body is seen after death – but the doctor must have attended during the last illness and not merely after the death. There is no 24 hour rule for patients who die in hospital, although some registrars question cases where there has been little time to assess the illness, or the patient had not been seen by a doctor for some time.

There are certain causes of death that some families find difficult to accept on a death certificate. The instructions given with the certificate books set out some acceptable alternatives. The expression senility can cause offence to some, but there is often no alternative, other than old age. Discussion with the coroner's office may help find lawful ways to avoid offence.

Stillbirths and neonatal deaths

The Births and Deaths Regulations 1987 provides special forms for use when certifying stillbirths and neonatal deaths. As with other types of certificates, the doctor must read the instructions and examples printed on the cover of the book of certificates. In the case of a stillbirth, there has never been a live existence separate from the mother. As the baby has not been alive to die, there is no need for a death certificate. Registration is with the registrar of births, stating that the baby was stillborn.

The form is completed by the attending doctor, but it can be completed by a registered midwife, if no doctor was in attendance. If nobody was in attendance who is qualified to provide a certificate, there can be a declaration from a person present at the birth.

If it appears to the registrar of deaths that the child may have been born alive or shown signs of life, then the coroner must be informed. Unfortunately, from the point of view of certification, every foetus is alive until it is born or dies. Even a tiny foetus that cannot have a separate existence, may make movements after a spontaneous abortion. There may have been attempts to resuscitate a baby born without a heart beat. This type of situation may give rise to confusion over which certificate to issue and many doctors, in any attempt to compromise, take the feelings of the parents into account in helping to decide which certificate to use.

The special circumstances of a neonatal death are also recognized in the 1987 Regulations. The death certificate to be used for a child that dies within 28 days of birth takes account of maternal diseases and conditions that may have played some part in the death.

Cremation

The most common form of disposal of a body is cremation. Where the death is not investigated by the coroner by post mortem or inquest, the doctor who certifies the death must also complete a comprehensive form for the crematorium referee. The body must be inspected after death. The referee is medically qualified and may seek further information before allowing the destruction of the body. In exceptional cases, there may have to be a post mortem examination of the body (Cremation Regulations 1930 as amended). In addition to the certificate from the medical attendant, the Regulations require a confirmatory medical certificate from another practitioner, who has been registered for at least 5 years and who is not a relative, partner or on the same hospital firm as the medical attendant. This doctor must have examined the cremation certificate from the medical attendant and also have examined the body externally. The confirmatory certificate is not needed in certain cases, e.g. where a hospital post mortem has been carried out by a suitably qualified doctor and the result of that examination is known to the attending practitioner, who has signed the form.

Completion of these certificates involves additional work and the BMA Private Practice and Professional Fees Committee recommends a fee for this work.

Removal of pacemaker

If the patient has a pacemaker, it must be removed prior to cremation to prevent an explosion and, once again, a fee is recommended by the BMA for this additional non-contractual work.

Removal of a body out of England or burial at sea

Removal of a body out of England or burial at sea removes the body from the jurisdiction of the coroner. The coroner has to be informed and will provide the necessary certificate, after due inquiry.

Donating a body for anatomical dissection

If a doctor is asked for advice about the donation of a body for anatomical dissection, the Department of Anatomy at the nearest medical school should be informed. If they do not need the body, they may suggest referral to the Inspector of Anatomy. It is unlikely that a body will be of use after a coroner's autopsy, although some organs and heart valves may be of use for transplantation. If the body is accepted by the medical school, they will collect it and will arrange for its subsequent disposal.

The family may want to organize a subsequent funeral; and/or participate in an annual memorial service held by the medical school for all those who have given their bodies.

The coroner

The coroner is a doctor or lawyer of at least 5 years' standing, and his district is related to a Local Authority area, (e.g. county area or a group of districts or boroughs). As described previously, the coroner must investigate every death where the body is lying within the district, unless the deceased person was attended by a registered medical practitioner, who attended in the last illness and who has delivered a certificate of death to the registrar of deaths, disclosing a natural cause for the death.

Where the coroner is informed that there is a body lying within his district that has died a violent or unnatural death, or a sudden death of unknown cause, the coroner must initiate an inquiry (Coroners Act 1988, Section 8).

Deaths are referred to the coroner in two ways. First, if a body is found or is brought into the district from overseas. Second, if a doctor has attended the deceased, but the death is not known to be from a natural cause. If the death is suspicious then the police may be involved.

When a death is referred to the coroner, there are three courses of action.

1 After inquiry the coroner may say that the death can be registered from the doctor's death certificate. The registrar of deaths is notified by Form A. If the disposal of the body is by cremation, the doctor provides the forms.
2 The coroner orders a post mortem examination of the body. If this discloses a natural cause of death, the coroner informs the registrar of deaths via Form B. If the family want a cremation, the coroner provides the form without charge.
3 If it has been impossible to show that the death was due to natural causes at the post mortem examination, the coroner must hold an inquest.

In 1990 there were 562,000 deaths reported in England and Wales; 180,000 of which were reported to a coroner. Coroners ordered 132,000 post mortem examinations and there were 22,000 inquests.

A post mortem examination

This is carried out in a hospital or public mortuary. In cases of suspected murder/manslaughter the coroner consults with the chief police officer and the examination is made by a Home Office pathologist. If there is time, the coroner informs the family, family doctor, Health and Safety Inspector and others of the time and place of the post mortem. The coroner's office will have tried to speak to any doctor who has treated the deceased, so that they know that the patient has died, and to obtain any information that may assist the pathologist. Unless the autopsy discloses an obviously natural cause of death, the coroner can order special examinations such as toxicology, histology and bacteriology tests, X-ray etc. (Coroners Act 1988, Sections 19 and 20)

The full written report of the pathologist may not be available for some time, but a telephone call to the coroner's office will give the immediate result. A stamped, addressed envelope, with a request, will ensure a copy of the report in most cases (The Coroners' Records (Fees for Copies) Regulations 1990 provide for fees, but the informal arrangement usually works).

Where a death is not natural, the coroner and police may be reluctant to provide a post mortem report before it is produced in evidence.

An inquest

The Coroners' Act 1988, Section 11 provides for the coroner to summon witnesses and to take evidence on oath. In order to know which witnesses to call, the coroner or the police may ask for statements from potential witnesses, and a doctor may be asked for a written report. There is a fee chargeable for this service. A doctor is not obliged to write a report, but it may avoid delays and the need to attend an inquest. Provided that nobody wishes to question a witness, a written report may be used in evidence (Rule 37, Coroners' Rules

1984). The duty of confidentiality to a patient does not apply to giving evidence to the coroner after death. Information that might assist the coroner to ask the right questions and avoid the wrong ones, may be given by telephone, if it is not desirable to have it read out publicly. (Symptoms may be caused by family problems and not by illness. Tact can often avoid unnecessary distress, without distorting the truth.)

An inquest is not a trial. It is an inquiry to determine who the deceased person was and how, when and where the death occurred (Coroners' Act 1988, Section 11(5)). A conclusion, such as 'accidental death' is usually appended to this. The coroner may sit alone or with a jury of 7 to 11 persons. Save in matters of national security, the inquest is held in public and the press may attend. Any person with a proper interest (defined in the Coroners' Rules 1984, Rule 20) may attend the inquest, question witnesses and be legally represented. This includes the family and any person whose conduct may be called into question. The possible need for representation of a doctor is discussed elsewhere, but in most cases, the medical evidence is needed to show that the death was caused by some earlier injury or disease, for example, few families have heard of pulmonary embolism.

Medical records

A doctor attending an inquest is advised to bring any notes and records concerning the deceased. The coroner can issue a subpoena to have them produced, but this is rarely used. If the conduct of a doctor is called into question, apart from being represented at the inquest, s/he is entitled to ask for a copy of the notes of evidence of the inquest, when the inquest is complete, upon payment of a statutory fee.

Inquests and other inquiries

If a person is charged with causing the death of the deceased, the inquest is adjourned and the death is registered. The criminal trial takes place and it is most unusual for the inquest to be resumed. Where there is a judicial or other similar inquiry into a death or number of deaths, the coroner usually awaits the outcome of that inquiry, before holding the inquest. This avoids duplication or omission of evidence.

Useful pamphlets

The Home Office produce a free pamphlet on *The work of the coroner*. The coroner's office will have copies for families who wonder why the coroner has to be involved and if it will delay the funeral etc.

The Foundation for the Study of Infant Deaths have pamphlets for the family who have lost a baby. There is no charge and, fortunately, a doctor will need few copies.

Citizens Advice Bureaux provide advice without charge. In sudden death, the family may be in financial difficulties and the bureau can advise whether legal advice will be rewarding.

What to do when somebody dies, produced by *Which* can help a family through this potential minefield at a traumatic time.

7 The Mental Health Act 1983

Edward Josse

Definitions

THE Mental Health Act 1983 provides the legal instrument (as did earlier Acts) which enables society to act in the interests of and on behalf of patients and those convicted of certain criminal offences who are diagnosed as having certain abnormal mental conditions as defined in the Act.

The relevant mental conditions are defined in the Act as follows:

1 '**Mental disorder** means mental illness, arrested or incomplete development of mind, psychopathic disorder and any other disorder or disability of mind . . .'
2 '**Severe mental impairment** means a state of arrested or incomplete development of mind which includes severe impairment of intelligence and social functioning and is associated with abnormally aggressive or seriously irresponsible conduct on the part of the person concerned . . .'
3 '**Mental impairment** means a state of arrested or incomplete development of mind (not amounting to severe mental impairment) which includes significant impairment of intelligence and social functioning and is associated with abnormally aggressive or seriously irresponsible conduct on the part of the person concerned . . .'
4 '**Psychopathic disorder** means a persistent disorder or disability of mind (whether or not including significant impairment of intelligence) which result in abnormally aggressive or seriously irresponsible conduct on the part of the person concerned.'

However, a person may not be dealt with under the provisions of the Act as suffering from a mental disorder purely by reason of promiscuity, other immoral conduct, sexual deviancy or dependence on alcohol or drugs. Clinical judgement has to be relied on. Clearly a patient has to be suffering from a mental disorder in order for the provisions of the Act to apply. Furthermore, the Act in Part II, Section 2, Paragraph 2(b) (repeated in other relevant paragraphs) states that a person *'ought to be so detained in the interests of his own health or safety or with a view to the protection of other persons'*. Additionally these grounds for compulsory admission are modified in the cases of persons diagnosed as having psychopathic disorders or mental impairment by the phraseology as set out in Part II, Section 3, Paragraph 2(b) that *'such treatment is likely to alleviate or prevent a deterioration of his condition'*.

Herein lie at least three problems. Firstly, a doctor should have regard to the psychosis-like effects, which may be short lived if diagnosed, seen clinically after the taking of drugs such as alcohol, corticosteroids and digoxin, or in association with certain physical disorders such as hypoglycaemia, cerebral tumours, various endocrine diseases or vitamin deficiency states.

Secondly, difficulties may arise in certain psychopathic conditions, which a psychiatrist feels do not fall within the terms of the Act regarding treatment but which, nevertheless, comply with the dangers to self or others.

Thirdly, it must be recognized that certain behaviour may appear bizarre and irrational but in itself may not provide grounds for compulsory detention if the health, safety and protection elements as set out in the Act are not compromised.

The Act also sets out the conditions under which a patient may be placed under a guardianship.

Some attempt, within the Act, has been made to clarify the grounds on which treatment may be given either with or without the consent of a detained patient in hospital but clearly not all scenarios have been covered. Patients detained under the 72 hour emergency situation (Section 4) or via a constable (Section 136) are expressly excluded from the treatment provisions (Section 56). It would still appear to be legally impossible to treat compulsorily detained patients under any of the provisions of the Act or those placed under a guardianship on an out-patient or community basis.

The 1983 Act places greater emphasis on safeguarding the rights of patients in relation to detention, treatment and access to tribunals. However, the underlying thrust of the Act builds on the provisions set out in the earlier 1959 Act. Unfortunately many of the section numbers have been altered in the current Act.

The GP is only likely to be involved in a small number of sections of the Act (unless he happens to be a doctor approved under Section 12, when his duties in this regard would not be that of a GP).

Section 2, Compulsory admission for assessment for up to 28 days (equivalent to Section 25, Mental Health Act 1959)

The 1983 Act specifies that an application under Section 2 may be made on the grounds that:

a the patient is suffering from mental disorder of a nature or degree which warrants the detention of the patient in a hospital for assessment (or for assessment followed by medical treatment) for at least a limited period; and
b the patient ought to be so detained in the interests of his own health or safety or with a view to the protection of others.

The applicant is either an approved social worker or the 'nearest relative'. The latter is defined in Section 26 in a descending heirarchy commencing with husband or wife and concluding with nephew or niece but regard is paid to the half-blood, illegitimate, common law or co-habitant status of would-be applicants. It is usually easier and emotionally more acceptable for an approved social worker to act as the applicant but consultation with the nearest relative whenever possible is required. Applications have to be made within 14 days of seeing the patient. Applications to a court may be made by an approved social worker (and by others specified in Section 29 (2)) if the nearest relative unreasonably objects to an application under the Act.

The application has to be supported by the recommendations of two registered medical practitioners. It is required that both shall have personally examined the patient and, if not together, not more than 5 days apart. Both must sign the legal instrument of recommendation on or before the date of the application. Of the two recommending doctors, at least one has to have been approved by the Secretary of State as having special psychiatric experience. It is also expected, where practicable, for one of the doctors to have been previously professionally acquainted with a patient. Clearly, this is likely to be the GP.

A medical recommendation may not be made by a doctor if acting as an applicant, a partner of an applicant or of the doctor providing another medical recommendation, an assistant of the applicant or the recommending doctor(s), if in receipt of or having certain financial interests in the maintenance of the patient or having certain family relationships with the patient, applicant or second recommending doctor.

After completion of the required legal formalities, a patient must be admitted within 14 days of the signing of the last medical recommendation.

Section 3, Compulsory admission for treatment – initially for up to 6 months

As in Section 2 the admission is founded upon an application and two separate medical recommendations. However, there are some additional caveats. If the patient's mental disorder is diagnosed as a psychopathic one or mental impairment, then the treatment available should have the likelihood of alleviating or preventing deterioration in his condition. Furthermore the written recommendations must state from which one or more of the four stated mental disorders the patient is suffering, the reasons why compulsory detention is recommended as opposed to voluntary admission and why other methods of treating the patient, if available, are not appropriate.

Section 4, Compulsory admission for assessment in cases of emergency – for up to 72 hours (equivalent to Section 29, Mental Health Act 1959)

An emergency admission materially differs from those in Sections 2 and 3 in that only one medical recommendation is required, which if practicable is given by a practitioner with previous acquaintance of the patient. The doctor need not be one approved by the Secretary of State under Section 12, but he must have seen the patient within the previous 24 hours by which time the patient must have been admitted to hospital.

The application may be made by the nearest relative (not any relative as in the 1959 Act) or by an approved social worker as in the previous sections within 24 hours of personally seeing the patient. The application has to state the urgent necessity for an emergency admission. Once admitted the application lasts for 72 hours unless a second medical recommendation is added as required in a Section 2 admission.

Once the legal formalities of the Act have been complied with, the applicant or his nominee then has the authority to convey the sectioned patient to a hospital within the time limit as set out described earlier (Section 6(1)a and b).

Section 135

A GP may be involved in one of two ways under this provision.

If a patient with a mental disorder has been, or is being, ill-treated or neglected in a place whether living alone or not, an approved social worker may under oath bring this to the attention of a justice of the peace. The latter may then issue a warrant authorizing a constable, who must be accompanied by an approved social worker and a registered medical practitioner, to enter the premises (if necessary by force) and remove the patient, if thought appropriate, to a place of safety for a period of 72 hours. During this time the usual compulsory detention provisions may be brought into operation.

Section 135 also permits a justice of the peace, on information received on oath, to issue a warrant permitting a constable to enter premises (if necessary by force) so as to remove a patient already subject to the various detaining provisions under the Mental Health Act to an appropriate place. Under these circumstances, the constable may but does not have to be accompanied by a registered medical practitioner.

Section 136

This is a special authority given to the police enabling a constable to remove a person suffering or apparently suffering from a mental disorder, in need of immediate care or control from a public place or one to which the public has access to a place of safety, which may be a police station or hospital for a period up to 72 hours. During this time a medical assessment could be made enabling further arrangements under the Act to be brought into operation if thought appropriate. It is at this stage that the patient's GP could be asked to attend the place of safety for this purpose.

Occasionally a patient's family doctor could be asked to examine one of his patients who has been admitted to a hospital under Section 4 or detained under 5(2) (for a patient already an in-patient in a hospital on a voluntary basis) in order to provide a second medical recommendation to permit longer detention under Sections 2 or 3.

Section 7, Application for guardianship

Section 7 has the effect of controlling the place of residence of a patient, compelling the patient to be put into a situation that enables medical treatment, occupation, education or training to be offered and compels him to allow access at the place he resides to any registered medical practitioner, approved social worker or other specified persons.

What the powers do not allow is compulsory treatment. There is no statutory right for the guardian to consent on behalf of the patient to treatment.

Under these provisions, the patient must be aged 16 years or more and be suffering from one of the mental disorders previously described, such that it is necessary in the interests of the welfare of the patient or the protection of other persons that the patient should be received into guardianship.

The applicant may be the nearest relative or an approved social worker, who must have seen the patient within the previous 14 days. The applicant has to be accepted by a local social services authority and the name of the guardian has to be identified.

The application has to be supported by two medical recommendations with one of the doctors being approved. They must have examined the patient together or within 5 days of one another. One of the doctors should, where practicable, have had previous acquaintance of the patient. This is likely to be the GP.

The other sections of the Act will be of little concern to GPs.

GPs are able to claim a fee for signing a medical recommendation (increased for an approved doctor). Usually approved social workers carry the necessary forms as claims are made through social services departments for onward transmission to the relevant Health Authority.

GPs and others involved in actions in pursuance of the Act are protected from any legal action unless any *act was done in bad faith without reasonable care*' (Section 139).

8 The Children Act 1989

Richard Williams and Jean Harris Hendriks

THE Children Act 1989 arguably *'brings about the most fundamental change of child law this century'* (White *et al.*, 1990), and it can be seen as a testimony to the rising status of children in Western Society. As the survival of children in Western nations has improved the focus of concern about them has moved towards developmental, behavioural, social problems and their abuse. As a consequence, there has been a gradual shift from the perception of children as objects to them as young people deserving of civil rights on their own account.

The aims of the Children Act 1989

The main aims of the Act are to:

1 bring together private and public law in one framework;
2 identify the rights of children in law;
3 achieve a better balance between the perception of children and the need to enable parents to be able to challenge state intervention;
4 encourage greater partnership between statutory authorities and parents;
5 promote the use of voluntary arrangements.

The principles of the Children Act 1989

The main principles embodied in this legislation are that:

1 the **welfare** of children must be the **paramount** consideration in making decisions about them;
2 the concept of **parental responsibility** replaces that of parental rights;

3 the ability of children to be parties, **separate** from their parents, in legal proceedings is **increased**;

4 Local Authorities are charged with duties to **identify** children in **need** and to safeguard and promote their welfare;

5 certain duties and powers are conferred upon **Local Authorities** to provide **services** for children and families;

6 **a checklist** of factors must be considered by the courts before reaching decisions;

7 **orders** under this Act should **not** be made unless it can be shown that this is **better** for the child than not making an order;

8 **delay** in deciding questions concerning children is likely to **prejudice** their welfare.

The scope of the Act

The scope of this Act is extremely wide and consequently it will have far reaching effects and major implications for the practice of all who work with or for children since it changes their standing in law, introduces new concepts relating to the responsibilities of adults, changes the structure and functioning of the courts and provides an entirely new range of Orders relating to the care of children in both private and public law.

The Act is arranged in 12 Parts to which are applied 15 Schedules. Particular attention is drawn to Part I which establishes concepts central within the Act, including the welfare paramouncy principle and that of parental responsibility. Part III gives substantial powers and duties to local authorities to ascertain children in need and to act in support of children and their families. This legislation also provides Regulations and Guidance with respect to children accommodated by statutory bodies and voluntary organizations and deals with private arrangements for fostering children as well as childminding and day care for young children.

The welfare check-list

When making decisions the courts are directed to have particular regard to:

1 the wishes and feelings of the child, taking into consideration the child's age and understanding;
2 the child's physical, emotional and educational needs;
3 the likely effect on the child of any change in his/her circumstances;
4 the child's age, sex, background and relevant characteristics;
5 any harm which the child has suffered or is at risk of suffering;
6 the parents' capacity to meet the child's needs;
7 the powers of the court.

Parental responsibility

The substitution of the concept of parental responsibility for that of parental rights is a change central in this law. The Act defines parental responsibility to mean, *'all the rights, duties, powers, responsibilities and authority which by law the parent of a child has in relation to the child and his property'*. Parental responsibility is given to both the child's father and mother where they are married to each other at the time of the child's birth. In the case of unmarried parents the mother is assigned parental responsibility and the father does not have parental responsibility for his child unless he acquires it. This is achieved either by application of the father to the court or the making of a parental responsibility agreement between the father and mother. It is clear that more than one person may have parental responsibility for the same child at the same time and people who have parental responsibility do not cease to have that duty solely because some other person subsequently acquires parental responsibility.

The new orders

Part II makes major changes in the orders available in family proceedings (private law) in which questions arise concerning the welfare of the children. The concepts of custody, care and control and access which have caused confusion and misunderstanding are swept away to be replaced by a range of new provisions. These orders are known as Section 8 orders.

Part IV concerns the new conditions relating to the making of care and supervision orders. The courts may only make such orders when satisfied that a child's circumstances are such that certain threshold criteria are met. Establishing these criteria, involves assessment of the child, his/her parents abilities and his/her circumstances according to a series of steps (Section 31).

Step 1 Is the child suffering, or likely to suffer, **harm?**

Step 2 Is this **harm significant?**

Step 3 If the **significant harm** suffered by a child is that of an effect on his health or development then how does his health or development compare with that which could be reasonably expected of a similar child?

Step 4 Is this **harm** or its likelihood **attributable** to the care given to the child or likely to be given to him if the order were not made?

Step 5 Is the **care** given to the child *not* what it would be **reasonable** to expect a parent to give?

Even if these criteria are satisfied there remains the further step for courts to consider which is that of showing that there are likely to be advantages to the child from making a care or supervision order which would not accrue if no such order were made (Section 1(5)). Healthcare practitioners may find themselves called upon, by virtue of their experience and training and clinical activities, to provide written, or to give oral evidence as to fact, or to express expert opinion on these issues.

Care orders are no longer available for children who fail to attend school or those facing criminal proceedings before the juvenile courts. The education supervision order is introduced for those who fail to attend school and as conditions of supervision the courts may order medical and psychiatric examination and treatment subject to the consent of the child, where s/he is deemed sufficiently capable of understanding.

Part V, which concerns the protection of children, introduces another new order, the child assessment order, and replaces the place of safety order with the emergency protection order. The place of safety order was an ex parte order, as is the emergency protection order, but rights of being heard by a court shortly after a successful application are afforded to parents by the emergency protection order.

	Children Act 1989 orders	Orders in previous legislation
Private law	Section 8 orders Residence Contact Specific issues Prohibited steps	Custody Care and control Access
Public law	Care order Supervision order Education supervision order	Care order Supervision order
Child protection	Child assessment order Emergency protection order Police protective custody	Place of safety order
Wardship	No longer to be used by Local Authorities as a route into care. May be available in exceptional circumstances only	Often used to gain the direction of the courts when care order application failed, not appropriate or result uncertain

Figure 8.1: Orders

Implications of the Children Act 1989 for healthcare staff

Partnership and co-operation

The major responsibilities arising from this legislation fall upon parents, others having responsibilities for children and upon Local Authorities. Nonetheless the Act has substantial implications for the NHS and for all healthcare workers who come into contact with children. One of the main themes of this Act is the encouragement of greater co-operation between those with responsibilities for children and the statutory and voluntary agencies. At least 18 Sections of the Act have implications for Health Authorities, Trusts and for health staff generally.

Section 27 enables Local Authorities to request the help of any other authority or person, including Health Authorities, in relationship to specified actions. These authorities are directed to comply with requests if this is compatible with their own statutory other duties and obligations and does not unduly prejudice the discharge of any of their functions. In the 1980s the Department of Health published, *Working together: a guide to arrangements for inter-agency co-operation for the protection of children from abuse*, and a revised edition, updated to take account of the Act and its Regulations and Guidance was published in late 1991.

Case conferences

This principle of partnership will have implications for informing parents and involving them in decision-making about their children. In many Local Authorities the involvement of parents in all or part of the proceedings relating to the reception of their children into care and subsequent reviews has become commonplace. However concern has been expressed about the extension of this practice to child abuse conferences. It is clear that if parents are to be involved in case conferences of this sort then particular attention will need to be given to the training of chairpersons and the way in which conferences are conducted. Many professionals have fears that important information might be omitted, that the proceedings might become acrimonious or that decisions will be inhibited and be made elsewhere. As a result many Local Authorities have adopted the procedure of having a portion of the meeting without the parents present to allow professionals to air their concerns in confidence. The Children Act is likely to bring greater involvement of parents in case conferences and also stimulate further exploration into their practice and effectiveness but, pending the outcome of such studies, the authors support the inclusion of a confidential portion of the proceedings.

Hospital in-patient treatment

Health Authorities and Trusts which intend to provide, or continue to provide, accommodation for a child for a consecutive period of 3 months or more are required to notify the responsible Social Services Department (Sections 85 and 86). In addition the Children (Secure Accommodation) Regulations 1991 extend the application of Section 25, which relates to the restriction of children's liberty, to children accommodated by the NHS who are not detained under any provision of the Mental Health Act 1983. The Mental Health Act 1983 Code of Practice is being amended as a result. Whilst this change is welcomed in principle the result might be the more frequent use of the Mental Health Act in child and adolescent psychiatric practice.

Consent

Consent has been defined as the voluntary and continuing permission of the patient to receive a particular treatment, based on adequate knowledge of the purpose, nature, likely effects and risks of that treatment, including the likelihood of its success and any alternatives in it (Department of Health and Welsh Office 1990). Consent is valid if fully informed and freely given by the person concerned. This applies to children as much as to adults (Jones, 1991). The Children Act endeavours to bring into statute several matters relating to consent which have been the subject of common law or decided by case law.

Section 3(5) of the Children Act provides that, '*A person who a) does not have parental responsibility for a particular child; but b) has care of the child, may, subject to the provisions of this Act do what is reasonable in all the circumstances of the case for the purpose of safeguarding or promoting the child's welfare*'. This is seen as enabling adults not holding parental responsibility for children to give consent for emergency medical procedures.

The legal ability of children under the age of 16 to give their own consent to medical or other health procedures was unclear until 1986 when it came under scrutiny in the Gillick case. The Gillick judgement reinforced previous practice arising from the Family Law Reform Act 1969, in which children of normal development, over the age of 16, were considered to possess the ability to give consent to medical procedures. It was particularly important in clarifying the position of children under the age of 16 who were also seen as capable of giving valid consent, if the individual was, '*of sufficient understanding and intelligence to enable him or her to understand fully what is proposed*'. If a child below the age of 16 was considered not to have this degree of understanding, parental consent or the consent of the person responsible for the child was envisaged as required. The Children Act and its Schedules recurrently require the child's consent to examination and treatment and allow him or her to refuse if s/he is, '*of sufficient understanding to make an informed decision*'. It is important to realize that the Regulations and Guidance to the Act place decisions into the hands of doctors as to the ability of children and young people to make informed decisions. Jones (1991) offers useful advice to practitioners on the issues which need to be considered in deciding whether or not a child is 'Gillick competent'.

Training and further reading

Particular attention is drawn to *The Children Act 1989: an introductory guide for the NHS* (Department of Health, 1991). It is free, available from FHSAs and provides a brief and clear summary orientated to the needs of healthcare practitioners.

Despite the growing number of explanatory texts, The Children Act document will remain the only truly authoritative source of information on what is or is not lawful in relation to children. The *Introduction to the Children Act* (HMSO, 1989) highlights the comprehensive nature of the Act and its aims and principles.

In 1991 the Department of Health published the detailed Guidance and Regulations in nine volumes. They are detailed and give authoritative guidance as to the intentions and requirements of the Act and allow a comprehensive picture of its potential impact on professional practice to be formed.

A series of explanatory texts on the Act have been published. *A guide to the Children Act 1989* (White, Carr and Lowe, 1990), contains a commentary on the main provisions and reproduces the Act in full. A number of statutory, voluntary and educational bodies have also produced training packs. These include the Open University, the National Children's Bureau and the Department of Health.

All practitioners are urged to take advantages of short training courses on the Act, which should be provided locally by Health and Local Authorities.

Early in 1992 the Royal College of Psychiatrists published *A concise guide to the Children Act 1989* (Williams, 1992). Whilst being a brief summary of the Act, it expands on some of the issues raised in this chapter and provides a 'page to view' commentary of each of the major orders which the Act has established. It is short (26 pages only) and is intended as a practical guide for use in clinical practice.

Bibliography

(1989) *Children Act 1989.* HMSO, London
(1989) *An introduction to the Children Act 1989.* HMSO, London
(1991) *The Children Act 1989: an introductory guide for the NHS.* Department of Health, London

(November, 1989) *The Children Act 1989*. No. 91. National Children's Bureau, London

(1991) *The Children Act 1989, Guidance and Regulations*. HMSO, London
Volume 1 Court Orders
Volume 2 Family Support, Day Care and Education Provision for Young Children
Volume 3 Family Placements
Volume 4 Residential Care
Volume 5 Independent Schools
Volume 6 Children with Disabilities
Volume 7 Guardians ad Litem and Court Processes
Volume 8 Private Fostering and Miscellaneous
Volume 9 Adoption and The Children Act

White, R, Carr P and Lowe N (1990) *A guide to the Children Act 1989*. Butterworths, London

(1991) *Working together: A guide to arrangements for inter-agency co-operation for the protection of children from abuse*. Department of Health, London

Jones D P H (1991) Working with the Children's Act: tasks and responsibilities of the child and adolescent psychiatrist. In: Lindsey C (Ed) *The proceedings of The Children Act study day*. Royal College of Psychiatrists, London

(1990) *Code of practice, Mental Health Act 1983*. Department of Health and the Welsh Office. HMSO, London

(1991) *Guidance on consent to management and treatment*. NHS Management Executive, London

Williams R (ed) (1992) *A concise guide to the Children Act 1989*. Gaskell, London

Acknowledgement

The authors have benefited from many informal discussions with colleagues and wish to acknowledge their assistance, especially that of David Jones.

9   The General Medical Council

John Fry

Why a General Medical Council?

THE Medical Act 1858 that established the General Medical Council (GMC) was the culmination of 20 years of bitter bickering among 19 licensing bodies, each jealous of its own authority, and pressure from the large number of unqualified practitioners fearful for their future.

Essentially the General Council of Medical Education and Registration of the United Kingdom was created to protect the public by ensuring standards of education and practice and protect the profession from the competition of unqualified practitioners.

Its main functions are to act as an independent body responsible for standards of undergraduate medical education, conduct, ethics and performance.

It is there because if it were not there, there would have to be a similar body to carry out the same functions, perhaps with less independence and more under government control.

What is the GMC?

The GMC has been established by Act of Parliament and its powers and duties are conferred and regulated by statute. It is under the jurisdiction of the Privy Council.

This means that it has certain functions that it must perform and carry out as directed by statute. It is not a body to serve professional interests and it must always keep the public interest in mind.

The GMC and the profession must realize, therefore, that Parliament can at any time change its functions and powers and even replace it with something else. The medical profession should realize that it is something to be treasured and protected because the alternative would almost certainly reduce medical representation and increase lay and political powers.

The GMC, at present, comprises 102 members (more than double the size of 20 years ago), Of these 54 are elected by the profession; 35 are appointed by universities, colleges and faculties; and 13 are nominated by the Privy Council (mostly lay persons). The reason why the GMC is so large is because there has to be a majority of elected members.

The Council elects its own President, for up to 7 years, who is its head. There is a lay staff of over 100 headed by the registrar.

It is pertinent to note that the 54 elected members are so elected every 5 years, but only about one-third of registered medical practitioners actually vote, a sad reflection on the perceived importance of the GMC.

How does the GMC work?

The full Council only meets 2 or 3 times a year. Most of its work is carried out through various committees and by its staff.

The committees are:

1 The **President's Advisory Committee** which has replaced a much larger Executive Committee and considers important issues and problems and reports to Council.
2 The **Education Committee** which is concerned with the undergraduate curriculum, the pre-registration year, additional qualifications and higher specialist training and co-ordination of all stages of medical education.
3 The **Registration Committee** which supports the complex process of registration. There are 140,000 names of doctors on the 'home' principal list, of whom less than 100,000 work in the NHS.

    Note: It is very important to notify the GMC of any change of address. Erasure can take place if repeated letters from the GMC are unanswered for 6 months.
4 The **Overseas Committee** which is concerned with registration of doctors who qualified overseas.
5 The **Committee of Standards of Professional Conduct and on Medical Ethics** which considers the ever changing old and new issues in these fields.
6 Professional conduct and fitness to practise is dealt with by three committees:

    • **Preliminary Proceedings Committee**

- Professional Conduct Committee
- Health Committee.

7 The **Finance and Establishment Committee** which is responsible for collecting and spending over £6 million a year to run the GMC.

Serious professional misconduct

The GMC is best known to the public and the profession for its disciplinary procedures and, most dramatically, hearings in which doctors may be 'struck off'. In fact, in 1990, out of 140,000 doctors on the Register in the UK, 13 were erased and 20 suspended.

Central to disciplinary actions is the possibility of a doctor being found guilty of *'serious professional misconduct'*. There is no easy definition of this statement. Each case has to be interpreted individually as to whether it may be *'conduct in a professional respect judged by the rules, written or unwritten governing the profession.'*

What happens if a GP is accused of serious professional misconduct?

Every year there are about 1000 complaints received by the GMC about doctors. They come from a variety of sources:

- convictions of registered medical practitioners (apart from minor traffic offences) are notified by the police to the GMC;
- the Department(s) of Health may notify reports of Medical Service Committee cases (of GPs) and Committee of Enquiry cases (hospital doctors) where the doctor has been found 'guilty';
- individuals complain to the GMC about doctors in relation to themselves, families or friends, or through public bodies such as Members of Parliament, Community Health Councils, FHSAs, District or Regional Health Authorities;
- doctors complain about doctors.

Each complaint is carefully scrutinized and dealt with via a formal procedure.

The first examination is carried about by the GMC staff in the division that is expert and experienced in the matter. They work to agreed rules and sift out those that are not within the statutory remit of the GMC.

The second step involves the preliminary screeners. These are doctors (3) and lay members (2) of the Preliminary Proceedings Committee (PPC) who are sent papers on all cases which cannot be dealt with by the staff. The possible decisions are:

1 no action, i.e. 'case dismissed';
2 referral to the whole PPC;
3 sending an invitation for the doctor to comment on the complaint, but with no further action likely to be taken, and if a doctor is 'sick' then health procedures can be instituted.

The third step is a hearing by the whole Preliminary Proceedings Committee. The PPC is elected by the Council and meets at least three times a year to take decisions on about 50 cases at each session. The cases are considered on the papers prepared by the staff. The PPC is advised by a legal assessor and solicitor who sit with it. Decisions can be:

1 no further action;
2 a warning letter of advice to the doctor;
3 postponement for further information;
4 referral to the preliminary screener for health by adjourning the case *sine die* for subsequent reports;
5 referral for a public hearing by the PPC when there is a strong possibility of serious professional misconduct;
6 in rare cases the PPC can order immediate suspension after a private hearing, where the doctor is considered a danger to the public.

The fourth step is a referral for a public hearing by the PPC. This committee is elected by Council and usually has three panels which meet a few times each year, depending on the number of cases. The proceedings are akin to a law court with counsel representing the doctor and the GMC. Hearings can be lengthy.

Possible decisions are:

1 conclusion of the case with no further action;
2 postponement for a further hearing;
3 conditional registration, that is the doctor is expected to take action to improve performance;
4 suspension from the Register for up to 12 months;
5 total erasure from the Register for an indefinite period;
6 referral to the Health Committee.

The doctor and his legal advisers can appeal against the decision.

Sick doctors

For sick doctors, there are health procedures. Where a doctor may be so sick as to be a danger to patients, his fitness to practise is referred to a preliminary screener for health who can request the doctor to undergo examination and report by two doctors nominated by the GMC, and one of his own choice. Their reports are considered by the screener who suggests care for the doctor and decides whether the doctor can continue to practise freely or with conditions attached.

If the doctor refuses to co-operate, then he is referred to a hearing of the Health Committee. This committee seeks to encourage the doctor to co-operate in treatment but, if he refuses, it has the power to suspend him from the Register (but not to erase him).

What types of serious professional misconduct are handled?

The Annual Reports of the GMC list the numbers of cases dealt with under various categories and the GMC Blue Book expands on these. They include:

1 Neglect or disregard of personal responsibilities to patients for their care and treatment which includes failure to carry out good standards of care involving diagnosis and treatment, neglect in proper examination, such as skimped or neglected history-taking or physical examination; failure to investigate by such simple measures as urine tests for possible diabetes; neglect in applying correct treatment or failure in following up patients; refusal or failure to see or visit a patient; and failure to organize the practice to proper standards.

2 Improper delegation of duties to nurses and others. With the growing involvement of nurses in general practice, care must be taken not to ask nurses to undertake duties for which they are untrained or not legally approved, for example, making diagnoses and giving certain treatments without adequate supervision.

Use of, and poor communication with and within deputizing services can lead to complaints.

3 Abuse of privileges, such as the issue of false certificates when patients are not seen or not sick; signing documents or making

out reports that are inaccurate; prescribing drugs of dependence such as opiates, hypnotics and amphetamines, except in the course of bona fide treatment; and questionable self-prescribing or prescribing for one's own family.

4 Abuse of professional confidence, such as discussing or giving information on a patient's personal or medical history to others. This may result from dealings with the patient's family, friends or employers.

5 Undue influence on patients, to gain in a will, financial gifts, loans or seeking to gain any advantages through relations with patients.

6 Sexual or emotional relationships with patients, or members of their families.

7 Personal misbehaviour highlighted by convictions for indecent or violent behaviour. These can result in actions by the GMC because of damage to the public reputation of the profession and possible danger to patients.

8 Convictions for drunkenness or driving when under the influence of alcohol or drugs.

9 Dishonesty and improper financial arrangements, such as defrauding the NHS by false claims; fee-splitting; owning and using nursing homes; accepting loans or gifts from companies to influence prescribing or other forms of treatment; and dishonest completion of clinical trial or other research records.

10 Advertising. Although there is a more liberal interpretation of advertising by GPs providing information on their services to the public, undue self-promotion and claims for special skills are unacceptable.

   GPs would be well advised to read the section of the GMC Blue Book dealing with advertising.

11 Canvassing and 'patient pinching'.

12 Disparagement of professional colleagues through blatant criticism to a patient, the public or professional colleagues.

Facts about complaints

Bearing in mind that there are 140,000 doctors on the Medical Register, the numbers of complaints received by the GMC is relatively small (*see* Figure 9.1).

Complaints received by GMC	1000
• Dealt with by GMC staff without any further action	250
• Referred and dealt with by preliminary screeners	750
• Referred to PPC by screeners	150
• Public hearing by PCC	55

Figure 9.1: A typical year

Recent trends

The recent pattern of complaints to the GMC about GPs has highlighted certain issues that should be heeded and prevented.

1 Failure to visit patients at home when requested is the most frequent issue referred to the GMC as a result of Medical Service Committee hearings.
2 Rudeness by a doctor is a frequent reason for complaints by patients – although not of itself amounting to serious professional misconduct, it does reveal strains in relationships.
3 Clinical errors due to incompetence can lead to disasters and complaints. For example, missed diagnosis of meningitis, diabetes, cancer, myocardial infarction or ectopic pregnancy.
4 Insensitive care in terminal illness can be a cause for complaint by families of patients with cancer who have been mismanaged by GPs at home.
5 Canvassing of patients is a symptom of increasing stresses in, and break-up of, practices.
6 Breach of professional confidentiality is a common complaint from an employee who has been dismissed as a result of a report given by a GP to employers.
7 Contrary to public impression, complaints about improper **sexual relations** with patients are relatively infrequent.

Practical points: do's and don'ts

General practice should be a professionally exciting and rewarding field of medicine. It is where a doctor can contribute much to the health and welfare of patients, who appreciate the care given.

However, as with most personal relations, it can lead to problems and difficulties. These can, and should be avoided, if the doctor practises with a proper degree of concern for all patients. Care for patients as one would like to be treated oneself.

- Don't be rude or aggressive.
- Don't refuse repeated requests for a home visit.
- Don't try to take dangerous clinical short cuts or neglect basic procedures.
- Don't discuss confidential matters.
- Don't drink and drive.
- Don't become *too* friendly with patients.
- Don't run risks with NHS claims or forms.
- Don't accept dubious gifts from persons who may influence your professional actions.
- *Do* read the GMC Annual Report, Blue Book and reports of your defence organization.

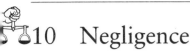

10 Negligence

Ralph Shipway

WHENEVER a GP agrees to attend a patient a contract is established whereby the practitioner has a duty to exercise reasonable skill and care. This applies whether the patient is accepted under the auspices of the NHS, on a private basis or if the treatment is being provided gratuitously. The scope of the contract is enlarged according to the specific agreement between doctor and patient and the GP always has a duty to his patient to provide reasonable skill and care of a standard such as would be provided by the majority of his colleagues.

What duty does a GP owe?

A GP owes a duty to his patient 'in tort', which is a civil wrong for which the remedy is an action in the civil courts for recovery of damages for an individual. The tort on which a GP duty to his patient rests is negligence and it defines the circumstances in which a duty of care arises and the standard of care required. It also governs the amount of damages payable by the negligent party in the items of loss which can be compensated when that standard is not reached.

What is negligence?

Negligence may, therefore, be defined as *'an omission to do something which a reasonable man guided by ordinary consideration would do, or doing something which a reasonable man would not do'*. It may immediately be seen that the GP is not to be judged by the standard of the consultant and need only display a fair, reasonable and competent degree of skill to attain the necessary standard of care.

Negligence is the breach of a legal duty of care owed by a defendant to a plaintiff which results in damage caused by the defendant to the plaintiff.

The Bolam test

The standard of care which has been the basis of the modern law of medical negligence was formulated by Justice McNair in the 1957 case of *Bolam* v. *Friern Hospital Management Committee*. The case concerned ECT treatment given to a patient suffering from depression and the action raised allegations that the doctor had failed to administer a relaxant drug before the electric shock treatment was given, had failed to control the plaintiff's bodily movements during the administering of the shocks, and had failed to warn the plaintiff of the risks inherent in the process. At that time trial was by jury, which is no longer the case, but the jury found for the defendants after the Judge had directed them on negligence as follows: '*The test is the standard of the ordinary skilled man exercising and professing to have that special skill. A man need not possess the highest expert skill; it is well established law that it is sufficient if he exercises the ordinary skill of an ordinary competent man exercising that particular art . . . Negligence means failure to act in accordance with the standards of reasonably competent medical men at the time . . . There may be one or more perfectly proper standards; and, if he conforms with one of these standards, then he is not negligent . . . He is not guilty of negligence if he has acted in accordance with the practice accepted as proper by a responsible body of medical men skilled in that particular art . . . Putting it the other way round, a man is not negligent if he is acting in accordance with such a practice, merely because there is a body of opinion who would take a contrary view . . . It is not essential for you to decide which of two practices is the better practice, as long as you accept that what the defendants did was in accordance with a practice accepted by responsible persons.*'

Prior to the Bolam judgment, Lord Justice Denning (as he then was) summed up the situation in the case of *Hatcher* v. *Black* in 1954 when he stated: '*Every surgical operation involves risks. It would be wrong and, indeed, bad law to say that, simply because a misadventure or mishap occurred, thereby the hospital and the doctors are liable. You must not, therefore, find the doctor negligent because something happens to go wrong as, for instance, if one of the risks inherent in an operation actually takes place or because some complications ensue which lessen or take away the benefits that were hoped for or because in a matter of opinion he makes an error of judgement. You should only find him guilty of negligence when he falls short of the standard of a reasonably skilful medical man.'*

If any doctor describes himself as a 'consultant' or 'specialist', it implies the possession of skills and understanding of the specialty beyond those of the ordinary GP and, by that implication, he is expected to use those superior skills. He has a duty to exercise that degree of skill and care which accords with his professional position so that anything less may render him liable to an action for negligence. Standards of care may vary in the light of further knowledge and what might have been acceptable some years ago might, in the present day, be unacceptable. The standard invoked at the trial, therefore, is the standard that is obtained at the time of the consultation or treatment and, therefore, is without consideration of developments in practice and knowledge during the interim between the incident and the trial. Again, Lord Justice Denning in the 1954 case of *Rowe* v. *Minister of Health* expressed the view '*We must not look at a 1947 incident with 1954 spectacles*'.

The Bolam decision has been reaffirmed by the House of Lords in a number of subsequent leading cases whether they concern questions of treatment, diagnosis, consent and disclosure of information, or in determining the best medical interests of the patient where a patient is mentally incompetent to consent.

Deviating from the norm

Deviation from normal practice is not, of itself, evidence of negligence, although it has been said that the practitioner who treads the well worn path will usually be safer, as far as concerns legal liability, than the one who adopts a newly discovered method of treatment. As long ago as 1767 it was stated that medical men cannot be permitted to experiment on a patient and ought not, in general, to resort to a new practice or remedy until its efficacy or safety have been sufficiently tested by experience. On the other hand, the courts will not press this proposition to a point where it stifles initiative and discourages advances in techniques and a line must be drawn so as to not to destroy inducements to progress. It must, however, be said that deviation from accepted practice is likely to result in a finding of negligence if the practitioner cannot establish a cogent reason for adopting the practice which he did.

Vicarious liability

The law may hold one person responsible for the tortious actions of another, even though there is no misconduct or blame on that person. An employer may be held liable for the torts of an employee, although a practitioner is obviously liable in law for his own actions and would be liable personally if found to have caused damage by negligence. The GP is not, of course, the employee of the FHSA as he is employed on a contract for services as opposed to a contract of service. Although the GP is, accordingly, an independent contractor, if he practises in partnership, his partners will be liable for the torts of a fellow partner and the liability of each partner for the other's negligence extends to the negligence of the partnership staff, including receptionists and those members of staff who provide auxiliary services.

What must a plaintiff prove?

A plaintiff bringing an action for negligence against a defendant must prove three matters in order to succeed in his claim. He must prove that a legal duty of care existed and that the defendant was so circumstanced in relation to the plaintiff that the defendant owed him a legal obligation to take care to avoid injuring him. This must always be the case when a patient initiates an action for negligence against a GP who has agreed to treat him.

The plaintiff must then show that there has been a breach of that duty by the defendant and that the defendant was negligent. As has been indicated, accidents can and do occur in the surgery and their happening may not in any way involve a lack of skill or care on the part of a practitioner. Lord Goddard in the case of *Chapman* v. *Rix* in 1960 stated '*No doctor is to be held liable for a mistake if he has used that degree of care that is expected of him and acted in accordance with a recognized practice*'.

The third essential factor for a plaintiff to prove is that damage has been caused to the plaintiff as a result of the breach. If there is no causative link between the negligent act and the injury suffered, a claim for negligence will fail. Even if a plaintiff establishes causation, to have a complete cause of action the damage alleged must be of a type of damage which the law recognizes as being recoverable, if it is considered as being of a type which is reasonably foreseeable as likely to flow from the injury and not too remote to be recoverable.

Breaking the chain

Has a supervening event occasioned by the plaintiff or a third party broken the chain of causation and thereby relieved the defendant of the consequences of his breach of duty? A supervening force which is held to break the chain of causation is known by the phrase *novus actus interveniens*. May there be a partial defence to an action for damages arising out of medical malpractice afforded by the doctrine of contributory negligence? The Law Reform (Contributory Negligence) Act 1985 provides that, where a person suffers damage partly as a result of his own fault, then the compensation received may be reduced in a proportion which the court thinks just and equitable having regard to his share in the responsibility for the damage. There is, in fact, no reported UK medical malpractice case where an allegation of contributory negligence has succeeded; no doubt reflecting recognition that patients often have little control over their treatment programme.

Res ipsa loquitor

There may be certain classes of injury or mishap where the mere fact of the accident effectively requires the defendant to rebut an assumption that they must have been in breach of their duty. The mishap may be said to speak for itself and of itself may be evidence of negligence. The rebuttal of such a prima facie case involves the defendant adducing an acceptable explanation for the mishap and, if no plausible explanation is forthcoming, then it is likely that the defendants will be held to have failed to discharge the onus upon them.

Failures

Whether the practitioner has fallen below the necessary standard of skill and care must depend upon the particular facts of each case and the precise circumstances giving rise to the allegations. There may be a failure in diagnosis, advice, or prescription.

Diagnosis is the basis of clinical judgement as it determines whether there is a need to treat and then to decide upon the mode of treatment required. In order that a proper diagnosis may be made, the practitioner must take a full history, conduct a proper examination and, where appropriate, organize tests, so that, if he fails to do this, he is likely to be liable for 'misdiagnosis'. If he fails to put himself in a position to make a reasonable clinical decision, then he will be found to have failed to provide the appropriate or necessary personal medical services of the type usually provided by general medical practitioners and, as such, will be found to be in breach of his Terms of Service. However, merely because a practitioner is found to be in breach of his Terms of Service, does not mean that a claim in negligence arising out of the same facts will succeed. A failure on the part of the GP to visit in response to a request may result in a 999 call and an immediate attendance by an ambulance resulting in admission to hospital. No damage will flow from the failure to visit but the breach of the Terms of Service may easily be established.

Consent

There must always be proper consultation and discussion before treatment and the GP must consider what he should disclose to his patient in relation to the inherent risks in the proposed mode of treatment. A patient must consent with full knowledge of the significant facts. Part of the practitioner's duty of care is to give advice and information to a patient so that the patient understands the nature of the proposed treatment. Just how much information a patient should receive must again depend on an individual situation. Should the curious be told more than the uninquisitive? The Bolam test is again of crucial importance as to whether the practitioner acted in accordance with the practice adopted by a competent body of medical opinion.

Negligent prescription may lead to liability against a practitioner. In 1989 in the case of *Prendegast* v. *Sam and Dee Limited*, the GP was found to be negligent with respect to poor handwriting which invited a misreading by a dispensing pharmacist causing the patient to suffer severe injuries because of the effects of the wrongly dispensed medicine.

Although a GP may, to a certain extent, rely on the diagnosis and advice given by hospital doctors when his patient is under the care of a hospital, there can be no abdication of the GP's responsibility and a failure to ascertain precisely what treatment the patient did receive in hospital may lead to negligence.

Records

The importance of clear and full records in relation to the defensibility of a claim in medical negligence cannot be sufficiently stressed. An action for damages for personal injuries must normally be brought within 3 years of the date of the accrual of the cause of action or, in the alternative, within 3 years of the date upon which the patient first had knowledge of material facts which could lead to proceedings being taken. If an action is initiated many years after the treatment, the presence of clear and efficient records will be of enormous evidential value.

The Access to Health Records Act 1990 came into force on 1 November 1991 and filled in a legislative gap in the network of legislation which gives individuals access to records kept about them. Health records kept on computer are accessible to the patient by means of the Data Protection Act 1984 and the Access to Personal Files Act 1987 gave individuals a right of access to records not held on computer held by Local Authorities and local Social Services Authorities. Health records had been excluded from the Access to Personal Files Act 1987 but, since the coming into force of the 1990 Act, the patient has a statutory right of access to their medical records, both private and those held under the auspices of the National Health Service. The Act is not retrospective and only provides for access to records made after 1 November 1991.

Expert opinions

Without supportive expert opinions a claim in medical negligence cannot be successfully defended. The criteria for contesting or settling medical negligence claims on behalf of a general medical practitioner are perhaps as follows:

1 clear and complete notes;

2 a clear and complete statement from the GP;
3 a GP who is prepared to go to court and who will present competently in the witness box;
4 the GP's own wishes;
5 supportive expert opinions;
6 the figure for which the claim can be settled and relationship to costs and possible quantum on loss at trial;
7 issues of principle.

The quantum of damage

Those reading about medical negligence actions in the press may react to the size of judgments and settlements with some confusion. Some awards may appear inconsistent with others. Some may appear disproportionate to the injuries sustained. In few cases is a breakdown of justification provided. Damages are a sum of money given as compensation for loss or harm of any kind and are intended to put the victim in the position he would have been in but for the accident, as far as money can. Damages are the pecuniary response the court awards for an actionable wrong done to the plaintiff by the defendant. The quantum of damage is the assessment in monetary terms of the value of that harm.

Lawyers analysing potential awards do so under various heads of damage, which are, principally:

1 damages for pain and suffering and loss of amenity;
2 special damages i.e. financial loss and expense already sustained by the time the case is disposed of;
3 damages for future financial loss and expense;
4 interest.

Certain of those heads are capable of more or less exact quantitative analysis but other matters are inexact and have to be assessed by the court. To a large extent, awards for particular injuries follow judgment tariffs which are comparatively easy to apply in the case of simple injuries but, a higher award must be made if an important leisure activity is destroyed, although a lower award might be appropriate if there was an exceptionally small life expectancy.

Greater difficulty in assessment is encountered when the symptoms are indefinite or where the prognosis is uncertain. Lawyers assessing damages rely to a considerable extent on the reports of awards for comparable injuries, upon their own experience and upon the experience of those with whom they work, and thus, have difficulty in rationalizing their advice to non-lawyers. Patients have already been in less than perfect health before being injured by their doctor's negligence so that which has to be evaluated is not a simple injury but the aggravation of a pre-existing condition.

In England, where awards are made by judges rather than juries, they are small by the standards of other countries but, as the value of money falls, the level of damages rises. Perhaps there has been some judicial reluctance to increase damages too much as huge awards against Health Authorities might limit their ability to provide medical services. However, awards must maintain a real value and frequently include damages for a miscellany of loss and expense incurred between injury and the conclusion of the case. e.g. loss of earnings, the cost of medical or nursing care, the cost of special equipment or clothing. The defendant takes his victim as he finds him and, if he injures a high earner as opposed to a member of the unemployed, this is quite simply his bad luck. The widely-held view that has been expressed is that it is all a rather elaborate lottery in which a few large prizes are awarded after a wait of several years. It has been put forward that there should be a system of no fault compensation for the victims of medical accident and the view was expressed in the House of Lords in February 1991 that the present tort-based system of compensation for the victims of medical injury is harmful, unpredictable and unjust.

Is moral judgement the right way to assess cases of medical negligence? Was the decision of the Government to pay compensation in the haemophiliac cases made because it was recognized that negligence was not the right basis on which to deal with this sort of case and that a wider humanitarian basis was correct?

Criminal negligence

It is possible for professional negligence to be classed as criminal if it incorporates such a degree of reckless and wicked disregard for the lives or safety of others that it amounts to a crime against the state. The negligence must go beyond a mere matter of compensation but be conduct deserving punishment. Could a failure to note warnings in the GP notes and to prescribe medication which had fatal results be regarded as being so reckless as to constitute criminal conduct? It is possible and, if those reckless acts resulted in the death of the patient, then a GP could be facing a charge of manslaughter, there having been total disregard of the duty of care the practitioner owes to his patient.

11 Confidentiality

Gerard Panting

Introduction

A doctor's duty of professional secrecy has been recognized as one of the most important elements in the establishment of trust between doctor and patient since ancient times. The Hippocratic Oath set out the basic principle in the fifth century BC. '*Whatever in connection with my professional practice or not in connection with it, I see or hear in the life of men, which should not be spoken of abroad, I will not divulge, as reckoning that all such should be kept secret.*'

Guidance for today's doctors is set out in the General Medical Council's publication *Professional conduct and discipline: fitness to practice* (The Blue Book), which is a code of professional conduct rather than a declaration on medical ethics. Doctors accused of breaching the code may face a quasi-judicial enquiry and if found guilty may be admonished, have conditions placed upon their registration, or be suspended or removed from the medical register. The General Medical Council's guidance reads: '*Patients are entitled to expect that the information about themselves or others which a doctor learns during the course of a medical consultation, investigation or treatment, will remain confidential. Doctors therefore have a duty not to disclose to any third party information about an individual that they have learned in their professional capacity, directly from a patient or indirectly, except in the cases discussed below*'.

The exceptions which must be discussed further are:

1 disclosure with the patient's consent;
2 disclosure in relation to the clinical management of a patient;
3 disclosure to a close relative;
4 disclosure to another third party in the best interests of the patient,
5 disclosure required by statute;
6 disclosure in connection with judicial proceedings;
7 disclosure in the public interest;
8 disclosure for the purposes of medical audit, teaching and research.

Finally the Council warns: '*A doctor who decides to disclose confidential information about an individual must be prepared to explain and justify that decision, whatever the circumstances of the disclosure*'.

However it is not just the General Medical Council to whom the doctor may have to justify his actions. Doctors also have a common law duty of confidentiality to their patients and the Data Protection Act 1984, and the National Health Service (Venereal Diseases) Regulations 1974 impose a legal duty not to disclose confidential information in the circumstances in which they apply.

Exceptions to the general rule of confidentiality

Consent to disclosure

A request for disclosure of medical records accompanied by a competent adult patient's consent poses little difficulty; armed with a valid consent the doctor is free to disclose the medical information requested.

However, problems may arise when parents seek access to their children's notes. A child below the age of 16 may seek medical advice and be able to give a legally valid consent to treatment to which the child's parents may object, the classic example being the provision of contraceptive services to girls under the age of 16 years. As a matter of good practice the doctor should attempt to persuade the child to discuss the proposed treatment with the parent or allow the doctor to do so on the child's behalf. If the child still refuses to involve the parents and has sufficient maturity and understanding to enable him or her to give a valid consent then the child is entitled to the same assurance of professional confidence as any autonomous adult. If the child is too young to give a valid consent, consent should be sought from the person with parental responsibility for the child.

Problems may also arise in matrimonial proceedings where child custody is at issue. The overriding principle here is that the child's interests are paramount and disclosure should only be granted with the appropriate consent and if it is perceived to be in the child's best interests.

The same principle applies when dealing with cases of suspected child abuse, if a doctor has reasonable grounds to suspect that a child has been abused the doctor's overriding duty is to the child and it is perfectly legitimate to supply reasonable information to the local Social Services Department or the appropriate officer of the National Society for the Prevention of Cruelty to Children.

Professional colleagues

To ensure continuity of care it is necessary to pass confidential medical information to medical colleagues and in some instances nurses, social workers and other professionals involved in the patient's care. However, disclosure should be limited to that which is necessary for the patient's care. The GMC holds the doctor imparting the information responsible for ensuring that all non-medically qualified staff are aware that the information has been passed in strict confidence.

However, what if information is requested by other medical or non-medical staff for administrative purposes such as the estimate of budgets for a fund-holding practice? The recipients of this information whether medically qualified or not are in no way participating or assuming responsibility for the clinical management of the patient and unless there is a statutory requirement for the doctor to pass such information on to a specific authority or the patient's consent has been obtained, such disclosure falls outside the guidelines laid down by the GMC and should only be released if anonymized.

The GP's Terms of Service set out specific instances in which the independent medical adviser on written authority from the FHSA may enquire about NHS prescriptions issued by the doctor and referrals to hospital services and other NHS facilities made by the doctor. GPs are also required to provide relevant clinical information to doctors employed by the Department of Health, the Welsh Office, the Scottish Office or Northern Ireland Office about a patient to whom the doctor has issued or refused to issue a medical certificate and answer any enquiries about prescriptions or medical certificates issued under the Terms of Service. Answering these enquiries is not dependent upon obtaining the patient's consent as disclosure of the information is required by statute – in this case the doctor's Terms of Service.

In May 1988 the GMC circulated a statement on the ethical considerations surrounding HIV infection and AIDS. It stated: '*The Council believes that where HIV infection or AIDS is being diagnosed any difficulties concerning confidentiality which arise will usually be overcome if doctors are prepared to discuss openly and honestly with patients the implications of their condition, the need to secure the safety of others, and the importance for continuing medical care of ensuring that those who will be involved in their care know the nature of their condition and the particular needs which they will have. The Council takes the view that any doctor who discovers that a patient is HIV positive or suffering from AIDS has a duty to discuss these matters fully with the patient'.*

On the specific issue of informing other health care professionals the Council stated: *'When a patient is seen by a specialist who diagnoses HIV infection or AIDS and a GP is, or may be involved in that patient's care, then the specialist should explain to the patient that the GP cannot be expected to provide adequate clinical management and care without full knowledge of the patient's condition. The Council believes that the majority of such patients will readily be persuaded of the need for the GPs to be informed of the diagnosis'.*

However, if the doctor's powers of persuasion prove insufficient he or she must weigh up the danger the patient poses to other healthcare workers against the damaging effect on the doctor/patient relationship if professional confidence is breached. If the specialist considers that other healthcare workers (including non-medically qualified staff) should be informed disclosure should be limited to the information necessary to prevent that person being placed at risk.

Relatives

The doctor who refused to offer any information to the relatives of the sick patient would seem callous in the extreme and traditionally doctors have been prepared to discuss the patient's illness with relatives to some extent. However, some care is required if complaints are to be avoided. The GMC advice reads: *'In exceptional circumstances a doctor may consider it undesirable, for medical reasons, to seek a patient's consent to the disclosure of confidential information. In such circumstances information may be disclosed to a relative or some other person, but only where the doctor is satisfied that it is necessary in the patient's best medical interest to do so'.*

What particular circumstances might lead the doctor to this conclusion? Shielding the patient from unpleasant diagnosis is likely to prove an insufficient ground unless the doctor considers that telling the patient is likely to cause serious harm to the patient's physical mental health (cf Access to Medical Reports Act 1988, Access to Health Records Act 1990 and Data Protection Act 1984 infra).

The GMC statement on the ethical problems associated with AIDS and HIV infection, considered the problem of the doctor's duty to the patient's sexual partner. It said: '*Questions of conflicting obligations also arise when a doctor is faced with a decision whether the fact that a patient is HIV positive or suffering from AIDS should be disclosed to a third party, other than another health care professional, without the consent of the patient. The Council has reached the view that there are grounds for such disclosure only where there is a serious and identifiable risk to a specific individual who, if not so informed would be exposed to infection. Therefore, when a person is found to be infected in this way, the doctor must discuss with the patient the question of informing a spouse or other sexual partner. The Council believes that most such patients would agree to disclosure in these circumstances, but where such consent is withheld the doctor may consider it his duty to seek to ensure that any sexual partner is informed, in order to safeguard such persons from a possibly fatal infection*'.

Disclosure to third parties

Disclosure to a third party in the best interests of the patient may exceptionally be justifiable even in the face of the patient's express refusal to such disclosure. Such instances are indeed rare but might occur where there was concern over the patient's capacity to make a reasoned choice and give a valid consent or was unable to act through excessive fear. It must be stressed however, that the general rule is that a patient's ban on communication with a third party is to be respected.

Statutory duty

In a variety of instances doctors are under a statutory duty to notify a particular authority of an occurrence such as a notification of infectious disease (*see* Figure 11.1) or a Notification of Drug Addicts under the Misuse of Drugs Acts 1971. Where a doctor complies with such a regulation the GMC will not criticize his action if a complaint is brought by the patient. Responsibility for notifying confirmed or suspected cases of food poisoning or an infectious disease rests exclusively with the medical practitioner attending the patient unless it is believed that another practitioner has already notified the case. Figure

England and Wales	Northern Ireland	Scotland
Acute encephalitis	Acute encephalitis/	Anthrax
Acute poliomyelitis	meningitis; bacterial	Dysentry
Anthrax	Acute encephalitis/	Chicken pox
Cholera	meningitis: viral	Cholera
Diphtheria	Anthrax	Diphtheria
Dysentery (amoebic or	Chickenpox	Bacillary dysentry
bacillary)	Cholera	Erysipelas
Food poisoning (all sources)	Diphtheria	Food poisoning
Leprosy	Dysentry	Legionellosis
Leptospirosis	Food poisoning	Lyme disease
Malaria	Gastroenteritis (person	Measles
Measles	under two years of age	Membranous croup
Meningitis	only)	Meningococcal infection
Meningococcal septicaemia	Hepatitis A	Mumps
(without meningitis)	Hepatitis B	Paratyphoid fever
Mumps	Hepatitis unspecified: viral	Plague
Ophthalmia neonatorum	Legionnaire's disease	Poliomyelitis
Paratyphoid fever	Leptospirosis	Puerperal fever
Plague	Malaria	Rabies
Rabies	Measles	Relapsing fever
Relapsing fever	Meningococcal	Rubella
Rubella	septicaemia	Scarlet fever
Scarlet fever	Mumps	Smallpox
Smallpox	Paratyphoid fever	Tetanus
Tetanus	Plague	Toxoplasmosis
Tuberculosis	Poliomyelitis: acute	Tuberculosis
Typhoid fever	Rabies	Typhoid fever
Typhus	Relapsing fever	Typhus
Viral haemorrhagic fevers	Rubella	Viral haemorrhagic fevers
Viral hepatitis	Scarlet fever	Viral hepatitis
Whooping cough	Small pox	Whooping cough
Yellow fever	Tetanus	
	Tuberculosis: pulmonary	
	and non-pulmonary	
	Typhoid fever	
	Typhus	
	Viral haemorrhagic fevers	
	Whooping cough	
	Yellow fever	
Notify: the 'proper officer' of the local authority who is usually (but not always) the medical officer of environmental health or consultant in communicable diseases of the local authority.	**Notify:** the chief administrative medical officer of the appropriate health and social services board.	**Notify:** the chief administrative medical officer of the appropriate health board.
Forms: available free of charge from the local environmental health departments	**Forms:** available free of charge from the appropriate health and social services Board.	**Forms:** available free of charge from health boards.

Figure 11.1: Notifiable diseases

11.1 lists notifiable diseases in England and Wales, Northern Ireland and Scotland.

Doctors who attend a person who they consider to be or have reasonable grounds to suspect is addicted to any drug controlled by the Misuse of Drugs (notification of and supplied to addicts regulations) Regulations 1973, are required to notify the chief medical officer at the Home Office within 7 days of the name, address, sex, date and birth and NHS number of the person concerned but no report need be made if doctors are of the opinion that the drug was required for the treatment of organic disease or injury or that the particulars have already been furnished by a doctor in the same general practice or hospital within the past 12 months.

Court orders

Lawyers are free to refuse to give evidence relating to their professional dealing with their clients but doctors do not enjoy this legal privilege and must release any information about their patients required by a court of law. Even if the doctor knows the court will force him to divulge his patient's secrets, no disclosure can be given until the order is made, at which point, refusal to comply would amount to contempt of court punishable by a fine or imprisonment.

Doctors subpoenaed to attend court should first decline to provide confidential information without the patient's consent on the grounds of professional confidence and explain their reasons to the court. But once formally ordered to respond to questions they may do so without fear of official censure.

Duty to society

Perhaps the most contentious exception to the general rule of confidentiality is disclosure in the public interest. The GMC states: '*Rarely, cases may arise in which disclosure in the public interest may be justified, for example the situation in which the failure to disclose appropriate information will expose the patient, or someone else, to a risk of death or serious harm*'.

Two common dilemmas for doctors are enquiries about patients from the police and the unfit driver.

In general, the police have no more right to confidential information than anyone else and no matter how forcefully their request is made, it should be rejected, unless the doctor is provided with the patient's consent or if satisfied the crime under investigation is of sufficient gravity to warrant disclosure, that the detection or prevention of the crime will be seriously prejudiced or delayed if material information is withheld and that the information will not be used for any other purpose and will be destroyed if no prosecution is brought or if it does not lead to a conviction. Establishing the importance of the information held by the doctor is most easily achieved by seeking an interview with the senior investigating officer who will have the necessary experience to appreciate the doctor's dilemma and the authority to give the assurances required.

There is one situation, however, in which a doctor is obliged to provide information in response to enquiries by the police. Section 172 of the Road Traffic Act 1988 requires that any person shall, if required, give any information which it is in his power to give which may lead to the identification of the driver. The case of *Hunter* v. *Mann*, 1974 (which concerned the identical section in the 1972 Act) established that doctors are not exempt from this provision. The doctor had refused to give the information requested by the police as he believed that such a breach of confidence could not be justified. He had however, advised two patients he had treated for injuries following a car accident that they should report it to the police. The court held that the wording of the section was clear and unambiguous and that the doctor was compelled to provide the information required.

Epileptics and patients who habitually drive under the influence of alchohol or drugs pose an ethical problem to their doctors. The duty to notify the licensing authority about medical conditions which affect an individual's ability to drive rests with the patient, not the doctor but in the knowledge that the patient presents a threat to other road users and pedestrians the doctor may feel unable to remain silent. If the patient refuses to respond to firm advice to stop driving, preferably in writing, the patient may be warned that if he continues to drive, the doctor may have no alternative but to report the fact to the licensing authority.

In the case of *W* v. *Egdell* and others, the Court of Appeal decided that a doctor who reported vital information to the appropriate authority was justified in breaching his duty of confidence to the patient as the public interest in protecting the public outweighed the public interest in maintaining confidences between a doctor and his patient. W had pleaded guilty to manslaughter after he had shot and killed five people and seriously injured two others. He was then detained in a secure hospital. Despite a recommendation that he be transferred to a regional secure unit the Home Secretary refused to consent to the move. Solicitors preparing W's application to a tribunal instructed Dr Egdell to examine him and produce a report in support of the application. In fact Dr Egdell concluded that W was more dangerous than had previously been thought and W's application was withdrawn. Dr Egdell subsequently learnt that this report had not been copied to the tribunal or the hospital and disclosed it to the Home Secretary himself. When W discovered what had happened, he attempted to sue Dr Egdell for breach of confidence but failed in both the first instance and on appeal.

Medical research, audit and teaching

The last exception to the general rule of confidentiality listed in the GMC's guidelines is disclosure of information for the purposes of medical teaching, research and audit. The GMC states: *'Medical teaching, research and medical audit necessarily involve the disclosure of information about individuals, often in the form of medical records, for purposes other than their own health care. Whereas such information is used in a form which does not enable individuals to be identified, no question of breach of confidentiality will usually arise. When the disclosure would enable one or more individuals to be identified, the patients concerned, or those who may properly give permission on their behalf, must wherever possible be made aware of that possibility and be advised that it is open to them, at any stage, to withhold their consent to disclosure.'*

Doctors who hold data about identifiable patients on computer and intend to use the data for research purposes should also ensure that their registration with the Data Protection Registrar includes this use.

If information about individuals including clinical photographs is to be published it should be anonymized or the consent of the patient obtained before the material is submitted for publication. Similarly, consent should be obtained before using the case histories of identifiable patients in lectures and other clinical presentations.

Armed forces doctors

Doctors in the armed forces are in the main in the same position as their civilian counterparts, but where a serviceman's condition poses a threat to the integrity of a fighting unit the doctor may consider the disclosure to the commanding officer is justified in order to protect the physical safety of the members of the unit as well as other persons. Despite the military setting the doctor must still be prepared to justify his action if challenged at a later date.

Occupational health physicians

Occupational health physicians have special problems in relation to confidentiality, as the primary objective of the consultation is usually to conduct an assessment of the patient's physical or mental health on behalf of a third party and often to submit a report on the individual suitability for certain jobs or even continued employment. Given the potential consequences of the consultation, it is imperative that the employee is in no doubt as to the purpose and consequences of the interview and that his consent to the examination is obtained at the outset.

The provisions of the Access to Medical Reports Act 1988 do not apply to occupational health physicians provided that they have at no time been responsible for the patient's care which in the context of the Act is 'conducting an examination, investigation or diagnosis for the purpose of or in connection with any form of medical treatment'. However, the provisions of the Access to Health Records Act 1990 and the Data Protection Act 1984, apply in full.

Disclosure of medical records to solicitors

In any legal action involving personal injury or death obtaining access to the patient's medical records is essential if the merits of the claim are to be evaluated. Consequently most solicitors make an early approach to the patient's GP requesting sight of the records. Whenever such a request is made two questions should be asked: who wants to know? and why do they want to know?

Provided that the request has come from the patient's solicitor or is accompanied by the patient's consent, the doctor can grant disclosure but in the absence of such consent requests from any other quarter must be rejected even if a doctor is threatened with a court order.

Very few requests for disclosure of medical records are made out of idle curiosity, legal proceedings are usually afoot and the nature of those proceedings may be of great relevance to the GP. In some cases it will be the GP himself who is the target of a possible medical negligence claim; if so he should inform his medical defence organization immediately so that correspondence with the plaintiff's solicitor can be taken up on his behalf.

Even where litigation may be contemplated against a doctor, it is usually appropriate to disclose the medical records as once the plaintiff has had the opportunity to obtain independent medical advice over 50% of claims are abandoned. In those cases where there might be some basis for allegations of negligence, withholding the notes for no good reason, merely protracts the proceedings for both plaintiff and defendant incurring unnecessary costs for both parties.

In cases where disclosure of the records is refused, either party to an action for personal injury or death may apply to the High Court for an order forcing disclosure. Under Section 33(2) of the Supreme Court Act 1981 (in England and Wales) any person who is likely to be a party to subsequent legal proceedings may apply to the High Court for disclosure of relevant documents, and under Section 34 of the Act any party to an action may apply for an order which compels a person who is not a party to the proceedings but appears to the court likely to have in his possession, custody or power documents which are relevant to a material issue to state if those documents are in his possession and if so to produce them.

The prospect of being served with legal proceedings compelling the doctor to disclose medical records may seem alarming, but in those instances where a patient refuses the opposing side access to relevant information, the doctor has no choice as he cannot disclose information about the patient without consent. However, once served with a court order the doctor may comply without fear of criticism.

Once it has been decided that disclosure of the records is appropriate, consideration must be given to the mechanics of disclosure. Many doctors have despatched original medical records to solicitors, and then found it almost impossible to retrieve them. This problem can be overcome by obtaining an undertaking from the solicitors either to return the records within a set period of time – usually 7 to 14 days or to accept photocopies and pay the doctor's reasonable photocopying and administration charges. Should the solicitor break this undertaking the matter may be referred to the Law Society for investigation. Original medical research should be delivered by hand or sent by registered post.

The Access to Health Records Act 1990

The Access to Health Records Act came into force on 1 November, 1991, a date of some importance as the legislation is *prospective* and only allows access to medical records written before that date if reference to an old note is required to make a current note intelligible.

The Act, which applies to England, Wales and Scotland but not Northern Ireland, established a right of access by the patient to whom the records relate and in certain circumstances other individuals. The Act also makes provision for correction of inaccurate records.

Under the Act a health record is any record containing information relating to the physical or mental health of an individual who can be identified from that information which has been made by or on behalf of a healthcare professional. The term 'healthcare professional' includes not only doctors and dentists but also opticians, pharmacists, nurses and numerous other paramedical occupations.

The very broad definition of health record under the Act includes not only the entire contents of the medical record envelope but also practice diaries and visit books although access to these can be withheld as disclosure would inevitably reveal confidential information about other identifiable individuals.

Applications for access must be made in writing to the record-holder and provided no addition to the record has been made within the previous 40 days a fee (currently £10) may be charged. Provided there is no reason to withhold access, the record-holder must allow the applicant to see the records within 40 days unless the most recent note has been made within 40 days in which case the time limit is 21 days. Should a copy set of notes be required the record-holder is entitled to charge copying and postal charges.

Applications may be made by the patient, someone appointed on the patient's behalf, in the case of a child the parent or guardian, a person appointed by the court to manage the affairs of an incapable person or after a patient's death by the patient's personal representatives or anyone who may have a claim arising out of the patient's death.

Access should be refused in a number of circumstances. If, in the opinion of the record-holder, disclosure would be likely to cause serious harm to the physical or mental health of the patient or any other individual or would reveal information relating to another identifiable individual that part of the record should be withheld.

In the case of children, the child's consent should be sought if the child has sufficient maturity and intellectual capacity to understand the implications of disclosing the medical records to the applicant. If the child is unable to give a valid consent the record-holder should only grant access if he considers it to be in the child's best interests.

The records of children, incapable patients and dead patients may be withheld if the record-holder believes that the information was obtained from the patient in the belief that it would not be disclosed to the applicant.

If following disclosure the applicant considers the record is inaccurate meaning incorrect, misleading or incomplete, he or she may ask for it to be corrected. If the record-holder agrees that there is an inaccuracy the record can be amended without further ado. However, if doctor and patient (holder and applicant) do not agree, the doctor is obliged to note the matters which the applicant regards as being inaccurate and where a correction or note is made the applicant is entitled to a copy of the amended part of the record free of charge.

Disputes over access to health records fall within the jurisdiction of both the county courts and High Court in England and Wales, and the Court of Session and sheriff in Scotland.

The Access to Medical Reports Act 1988

The Access to Medical Reports Act 1988 establishes an individual's right of access to medical records prepared for employment or insurance purposes, by doctors who either are, or have been, responsible for that person's care. The Act only applies to England, Wales and Scotland but similar provisions now apply in Northern Ireland under the Access to Personal Files and Medical Reports (Northern Ireland) Order 1991.

At the same time that the patient's consent to the preparation of a report is obtained, the commissioning company is required to inform the individual of his or her rights under the Act and to enquire if access to the medical report is required. This information is then passed on to the doctor.

If access to the report is required the doctor must allow the patient 21 days in which to make suitable arrangements to view the report. Patients who initially declined the opportunity of access may make an application to see the report up until the time it is despatched to the company and if so, must be allowed 21 days to make suitable arrangements with the doctor.

Once the patient has seen the report, he or she may agree to the despatch of the report unaltered, request the correction of factual inaccuracies or where the doctor declines to make the requested correction append a statement of his own or refuse to allow the report to be released altogether.

The patient is also entitled to a copy of the report for which a reasonable fee may be charged for being supplied with a copy. When a report is supplied the doctor must retain a copy for 6 months during which time the patient may apply for access subject to the exemptions below.

There are a number of circumstances in which a doctor may refuse his patient access to the report, but if so the report cannot be supplied without the patient's consent. The exemptions to access are where the doctor considers that allowing the patient to see the report is likely to cause serious harm to the physical or mental health of an individual or disclose information about another identifiable person (who is not a healthcare professional) in the absence of that person's consent or where disclosure would reveal the doctor's intentions in respect of that individual.

Disputes over access fall within the jurisdiction of the county court in England, Wales and Northern Ireland or the sheriff in Scotland.

The Data Protection Act 1984

Doctors who record information relating to identifiable living individuals on computer must ensure that they comply with the provisions of the Data Protection Act 1984. The Act applies to England, Wales, Scotland and Northern Ireland.

The Data Protection Act is based on eight principles (*see* Figure 11.2) and is designed to ensure that information relating to an individual is obtained fairly, kept up to date and stored securely. The individual whose data are stored (the data subject) has rights of access enabling him to check the accuracy of the information. The data protection registrar and the courts are empowered to require correction of inaccurate material if it is not undertaken voluntarily by the data user. Compensation may be sought through the courts if the data subject suffers financial loss as a result of inaccurate information.

1 Personal data shall be obtained and processed fairly and lawfully.

2 Personal data should be held for only one or more specified lawful purposes.

3 Personal data held for any purpose shall not be used or disclosed in any matter incompatible with that purpose.

4 Personal data held for any purpose shall be adequate, relevant and not excessive in relation to that purpose.

5 Personal data should be accurate and where necessary up to date.

6 Personal data held for any purpose shall not be kept longer than necessary.

7 An individual should be entitled at reasonable intervals without undue delay or expense:
  • to be informed by any data user whether he holds personal data relating to that individual
  • to have access to any such data held by the data user
  • to have such data corrected or erased where appropriate.

8 Appropriate security measures should be taken against:

  • unauthorized access to or alteration, disclosure or destruction of personal data
  • accidental loss or destruction of personal data.

Figure 11.2: Data protection principles

All data users who record data relating to identifiable living individuals must be registered under the Data Protection Act. Applications for registration should be addressed to: The Office of the Data Protection Registrar, PO Box 66, Wilmslow, Cheshire SK9 5AX.

In the first instance the applicant will be supplied with a Data Protection Act registration pack containing the application forms, an explanatory booklet, a return envelope and two address labels. All applicants must complete the part A form which has questions on general administrative details and a separate part B form for each purpose for which the data will be used. The part B form deals with the purpose of holding the data such as provision of healthcare, personnel/employee administration or statistical analysis.

Apart from dealing with registration the data protection registrar supervises the Data Protection Act. His office receives over 2000 complaints a year and if he finds that a data user is contravening the Data Protection Act he may serve an enforcement notice requiring that person to comply. In extreme circumstances a deregistration notice may be served. The data protection registrar may also prohibit the transfer of information outside the United Kingdom. Data users may appeal against the data protection registrar's decision to the Data Protection Tribunal.

Any individual is entitled to be informed by the data user whether the data held include personal data relating to that individual. The individual is also entitled to be supplied with a copy of the information relating to him that is held on the computer. The request must be made in writing and the data user is obliged to supply the information only after payment of a fee for access has been paid.

The medical context of the individual's right of access to information held about him or her has been modified by the Data Protection (Subject Access Modification) (Health) Order 1987. This allows information to be withheld from an individual if the data are likely to cause serious harm to his or her mental or physical health or discloses the identity of another person other than the healthcare professional. A doctor who withholds information must be prepared to justify his or her actions in a court if challenged at a later date.

Under the Data Protection Act individuals who suffer damage as a result of inaccurate data, loss of data or unauthorized disclosure of data are entitled to compensation for that damage and for any distress they have suffered. As yet there have been no claims for damages under the Data Protection Act but experience in countries where similar legislation has been in force for some years shows that litigation follows as the population becomes aware of its rights.

Doctors will be vulnerable if inaccurate or misleading information is retrieved from the computer and submitted in a report for legal, insurance or employment purposes. A patient who is turned down for a job, or suffers any other kind of loss due to disclosure of inaccurate data could bring a claim under the Data Protection Act without the need to prove negligence. Such an action could be defended on the grounds that sufficient care had been taken in all the circumstances as was reasonably required to ensure the accuracy of the data at the material time. Similarly, in claims relating to loss, destruction or inappropriate access, the action could be defended on the grounds that reasonable care was taken to prevent such loss.

Any person who regards the entry on a computer about him or her to be incorrect or misleading may apply to the court for rectification or erasure of the data, in addition to seeking compensation for any damage, loss or distress.

Section 5 of the Data Protection Act makes it a criminal offence for any person to hold personal data on a computer without being registered with the data protection registrar and once registered for anyone to obtain, hold or disclose any personal data unless that particular use is being declared on the data user's registration forms. Currently the commonest problem is a failure to reregister after expiry of the initial 3-year registration period.

12 Doctors and the police

David McLay

MOST doctors would prefer not to give evidence in court or to the police. However, there are medicolegal consequences from almost all acts of modern general practice. The fear of cross examination is an understandable one, but careful preparation can put the doctor in a strong position.

Doctors should be guided by the principle that a record made at the time of the observation, examination, test or treatment has high evidential value. Such records form the contemporaneous notes on which written and oral evidence depend. The definition of contemporaneous is usually thought to extend to 'as soon as practicable' after the event. No attempt should ever be made to pretend that notes are contemporaneous when they are not. If, for any reason, a note or record has to be amended, it should be done clearly, without erasure and the alteration should be initialled and dated. Careful, legible notes provide a solid basis for reporting; a scrappy, scribbled couple of words on a loose sheet invite accusation of sloppiness in thought and deduction. Notes cannot always be in a logical order, but statements and reports ought to be put in paragraphs, each following on from the preceding one.

Court hearings inevitably take place long after the incident or the circumstances giving rise to the dispute (in civil cases) or the offence (in criminal cases). For that reason, the court must rely on what is available as best evidence. Legal systems develop a body of law to regulate what is and what is not admissible to assist the court in understanding the dispute or offence. The oath or affirmation to tell 'the truth, the whole truth and nothing but the truth' binds a witness not to lie, but leaves room for the parties' representatives and the bench to judge how that truth emerges. In both litigation and criminal cases where medical matters are adduced, the issue concerns a biological entity that heals and modifies with the passage of time. Accurate description, supplemented as appropriate by illustration and the results of laboratory investigation, provide the best, indeed the only, possible substitute for the court's direct knowledge of the circumstances. Any description is given greater credence by the inclusion of measurements, preferably in both metric and imperial units. Clinical photographs are often of great value, but only when taken by a competent photographer able to recount details of lighting, film speed, exposure and colour rendition.

The doctor's own notes may be as technical as necessary, but reports or statements ought to be provided in a form understandable to a lay readership. Technical terms need not be avoided, but should be explained or put in parenthesis after the everyday description. A well compiled statement, which leaves no loose ends, is more likely to be accepted at its face value by the court. An all too frequent reason for personal attendance to give sworn evidence is simply to elucidate what a measure of forethought would already have made plain. These are simple admonitions, but doctors who often appear in court acknowledge why their expertise is often called upon: the paucity of observation and the appalling state of so many clinical records give rise to more questioning than any ignorance or negligence displayed by the practitioner who had clinical contact with the patient, witness or accused.

Disclosure

Patients reveal clinical information in the course of professional contact with a doctor in the expectation that confidentiality will be preserved. That confidentiality is for the benefit of the patient, not the doctor. Disclosure of such information is perfectly proper, therefore, at the patient's behest, for example in support of a claim to the Criminal Injuries Compensation Board.

The doctor/patient relationship

Does a normal doctor/patient relationship exist when the doctor is acting for an employer, an insurance company or the police? The purpose of these contacts is usually to bring professional skills to bear on the principal's behalf. The doctor has a duty to ensure that the examinee understands this clearly and is aware that a report is to be made, based on an examination. Even in the midst of such contacts, the examinee's status may revert to that of patient or matters raised may require referral to the patient's own doctor; a nice balance of judgement must then be exercised by the practitioner. The only truly privileged relationship is that between a client and his legal representative; the doctor is not absolved from disclosure on the direction of a judge – he or she is in contempt for any failure to comply. Having said that, judges can be depended upon to require an answer only when the information thus revealed is essential to a complete understanding of the point before the court.

The General Medical Council (GMC) has recently revised its guidance on professional confidence, but in many respects, the document is striking for what it does not say. For example, in the paragraphs relating to judicial proceedings, no overt advice is given to doctors who find themselves cast as witnesses in criminal enquiries. The GMC does authorize disclosure of information by '*a doctor summoned to assist a Coroner, Procurator Fiscal or similar officer either at an inquest or when the need for an inquest is being considered*'. Nevertheless, a doctor has a duty to object to disclosure when this would reveal confidential information about third parties. In practice, the initial inquiries into sudden deaths are made by police officers or by coroners' officers; it is obstructive to decline to disclose information to them, unless the considerations set out in the last sentence apply.

Guidelines have been agreed between the Central Consultants' and Specialists' Committee of the BMA and the British Association for Accident and Emergency Medicine on the one hand and the Association of Chief Police Officers (ACPO) on the other for doctors in accident and emergency departments who may be asked for non-clinical information about patients by police officers. In general, release of information without consent is held to be justified when there is an allegation that a serious arrestable offence (as defined in the Police and Criminal Evidence Act 1984, known as PACE) has been committed which will result in serious harm to the security of the state or to public order, serious interference with the administration of justice or the investigation of the case, death or serious injury or substantial financial gain or serious financial loss. These statutory provisions are echoed, albeit faintly, in the GMC guidance (disclosure in the public interest). Officers are also entitled to information assisting them in an identification of drivers who have committed some offences under the Road Traffic Act 1972.

The situations referred to above suggest that the request for information ought to come from an officer of at least inspector rank (this notion probably arises from the need, under PACE, for an inspector to authorize the taking of non-intimate samples from detainees). How far these considerations should move GPs when asked for information must remain for each to decide in the light of the circumstances of the case. The unsatisfactory state of the law on disclosure in the United Kingdom – with the few specific exceptions mentioned – is not mirrored everywhere; in some countries legal provisions require doctors to disclose information in defined circumstances or else indemnify those who do. Where the correct balance lies between the proper demands of the state as guardian of law and order and the obligations a doctor has to the patient may be an interesting question of theory, but when embroiled in a case, the practitioner must depend on conscience first, then on the defence bodies which have long experience of these dilemmas.

The Children Act 1989 introduces profound changes in the way society must treat children within a family. Emphasis is placed on the obligations of parents, other carers and society at large, rather than on their rights over children. Even court orders for assessment or examination will not be enforced against the objections of the child. In a similar way, the Social Work (Scotland) Act 1968 affected the whole approach to the statutory care of children and the view taken of them within the legal system. The implication that, in the context of any medical relationship, the doctor's duty is to the child (unless, of course, in reporting to a court or other authorized agency) reinforces the view that children, not their parents, are the patients. Information gained at an examination, if it gives rise to suspicion of abuse, in a physical or a sexual sense, must be clearly recorded, then shared with another practitioner, the police or social worker, as appropriate.

In the case of adults, suspicion of assault, physical or sexual, within a family must be discussed sympathetically but resolutely with the patient. It is the patient who has to take the decision about disclosure to the authorities. Many allegations of rape, some incestuous, are made in the context of a family planning clinic; there, too, the victim's own wishes must be respected, unless mental subnormality obliges the doctor to take active steps for the patient's protection.

Police organization

Within limits imposed by government circulars and the law, chief constables have a free hand to run their force (constabulary) in an operational sense, but depend for finance on the police authority. Half of any approved expenditure comes from central government sources. Chief constables, their deputies and assistants, together with certain Metropolitan Police officers, form the Association of Chief Police Officers (ACPO), which has the difficult task of advising the Home Office and their own members on policy and good practice, as well as representing the officers themselves in such matters as pay negotiations. A separate ACPO performs the same functions in Scotland. All police forces are subject to periodic review by HM Inspectors of Constabulary, whose reports are now to be published. Where inspection could become supervision remains a sensitive issue, both in the police service itself and to those who believe that local, rather than central, control should remain a feature of policing in Britain.

Beat officers are the backbone of the police service in the sense that they are visible, they provide the immediate contact with the public, they respond to calls in their area and they have to make themselves familiar with all the local occurrences of interest to the police. Some specialized departments which practitioners may often deal with are also usually staffed by uniformed officers, but local organization and functional responsibility vary from force to force. The community involvement branch deals with school and community liaison; their officers will be encountered at child abuse case conferences. Most forces have specialized child protection officers, and sexual offences units which deal with both men and women. The duties of traffic departments are obvious.

The coroners' officers to be found in large towns deal with deaths reported to the coroner or to the police, as do beat constables or inquiry officers elsewhere. Suspicious deaths and other serious matters also involve plain clothes detectives of the criminal investigation department (who still, as appropriate, must report to the coroner).

After a suspect has been charged, the conduct of criminal proceedings in the courts in England, Wales and Northern Ireland is now the responsibility of the Crown Prosecution Service; in Scotland, the procurator fiscal is responsible for both investigation (in which he has power to direct the police) and prosecution (his responsibility extends to any enquiry into sudden, unexpected death).

Written evidence

In England, Wales and Northern Ireland, evidence gathered by the police for the purposes of prosecution is usually taken as a statement.

Statements are formal documents, governed by the Criminal Justice Act 1967 and the Magistrates Court Rules 1968. After preliminary details of identification, the following paragraph is signed, '*This statement (consisting of . . . pages each signed by me) is true to the best of my knowledge and belief and I make it knowing that, if tendered in evidence, I shall be liable to prosecution if I have wilfully stated in it anything which I know to be false or do not believe to be true*'.

The doctor should retain a copy of any such statement, together with the notes and other documents on which the statement is based, so that all may be available to take to court. In court, it is routine to seek the bench's permission to use the contemporaneous notes to refresh the witness's memory. One effect of using them is that these notes will then come under scrutiny by the court and lawyers on both sides. To repeat what has already been said, any discrepancy detected between the original information and the facts and opinion given in the statement discredits the witness. Doctors are classified as professional witnesses, which implies that they may be asked to interpret their clinical findings or laboratory results within their expected area of knowledge; they are not, unless specially qualified, giving expert evidence.

The statement should begin with a recitation of the doctor's qualifications, position and relevant experience. The signatory's address appears on the statement, and it may be revealed in open court. The place and time of examination must be stated, with names of those present. It is helpful to capitalize the examinee's name whenever it appears in the statement. The more orderly the arrangement of the paragraphs in the statement, the more value it has to the court and the simpler the doctor will find time spent in the witness box, if called to give evidence.

Sometimes in England, and invariably in Scotland, a statement is taken down in writing by the inquiry officer, and (suitably transcribed) submitted as one of the case papers. Doctors are better advised, certainly in a complex case, to compile a formal report, for this will become a documentary production at any proceedings, when the witness is able to refer to it in answer to questions. The preamble should set out the identity of the person or official who requested the report, details of the examinee's name, date of birth and address. Consent for examination should be recorded, with a note of who was present during examination. If the report is based on a series of patient contacts, they should either be set out in chronological order, or the history and examination findings given separately. The opinion or conclusion precedes the signature, qualifications and post held. Each page must be signed at the bottom. Do not be tempted to an opinion which cannot be supported under cross-examination; if several explanations are feasible, say so.

Injuries[1]

In describing a lesion, it should be remembered that the provisions of the Offences Against the Person Act 1861 (an Act not applicable in Scotland) characterize wounds as arising from the destruction of a bodily surface, including mucous membranes; it does not matter how superficial the damage is, nor how small the area involved. Thus, somewhat sterile arguments arise over definition, but it is accepted that, although some abrasions may be wounds, contusions cannot be.

Lesions possibly arising from applied violence which come to a GP's attention include the following.

Erythema

Confusion arises when the reddening is part of a blush reaction, perhaps in response to embarrassment at examination, or is caused simply by pressure against a chair back. Skin affected by a weal is swollen, and sometimes pale rather than red; weals are seen after a thrashing as well as being a manifestation of skin sensitivity. Reddening or weals demonstrating the pattern of a beating with hands or an instrument do not persist beyond a few hours. For that reason, such marks are not consistent with a history of infliction several days before. It should not be forgotten that erythema is also a consequence of inflammation not associated with trauma. When seen near, upon or within the genitalia or anus the greatest care must be taken before assuming sexual abuse to be the cause (see page 130). In young girls, the internal skin of the vulva is not keratinized and is but a few cells thick, so allowing the vascularization to shine through.

[1]These are fully described in McLay W D S (Ed) (1990) *Clinical forensic medicine*. Pinter Publishers, London.

Petechiae

Rupture of minute vessels is caused by blows, traction on clothes, pinching, sucking and asphyxia. Some of these mechanisms will have innocent explanations. The lesions are, at times, very sparse and difficult to see without careful observation and good illumination. Do not forget to look for them in the mouth and on the conjunctivae. Petechiae coalesce into ecchymoses, but there is no satisfactory definition of those intermediate lesions.

Bruises

Contusions first appear where the violence is applied, but tend to spread locally and along tissue planes. Being caused by extravasated blood, swelling felt on gentle palpation is to be expected. Rather lighter, recent bruising is often more helpful in demonstrating any pattern which identifies a weapon. An example of such identification is the double line of bruising enclosing central pallor so characteristic of a single blow with a rod.

Abrasions

Unless very deep, these give a good indication of the type of surface causing the abrasion, and the direction in which force was applied. Unexpected surfaces, such as carpets, are capable of inflicting abrasions. Finger nails and teeth both leave characteristic patterns. Interpretation of the latter is best left to an odontologist.

Lacerations

Very deep abrasions are indistinguishable from lacerations, a characteristic of which is irregularity, except where they are caused by a blow to skin over a bony prominence. Lacerations of the scalp, for instance, must be examined minutely before they can be categorized confidently.

Incisions

These are caused by sharp instruments, but the wound itself may be multiple and irregular, depending upon the qualities of the skin involved. Stab wounds, also caused by sharp instruments, are unlikely to come to a GP's attention, certainly soon after infliction.

Burns

In non-accidental injury cases, cigarette burns and scalds are common. Some burns are the result of chemical, rather than thermal, damage.

Site and extent

Having established the type of lesion under inspection, it is essential to record its size and exactly where it is. Most anatomical features are duplicated on the other side, so allowing ready comparison, but a failure to record the affected side, the aspect of the limb injured, to distinguish leg from thigh, medial from median, are signs of carelessness that will be spotted in court. A flexible tape makes measurement simpler; not only should the dimensions be recorded, but also the distance from a fixed anatomical feature, such as the upper end of the sternum. If lesions are multiple, simple sketches with numbers referring to the written description are helpful both as an *aide-mémoire* to the witness before giving evidence, and to those who may be preparing a case.

Genital and anal injuries

All the forms of injury already mentioned are to be found in cases of sexual assault. In addition, the significance to be placed on infections, such as thrush, gonorrhoea, genital warts, and on other phenomena, such as anal fissures, the so-called reflex anal dilatation and the diameter of the opening in the hymen require very careful assessment; these signs remain highly contentious as pointers to diagnosis. There is considerable controversy about the aetiology of genital warts and their relationship to warts elsewhere. It is probably unsafe, therefore, for any practitioner who is not accustomed to examining possible sexual assault to give an opinion. Both police officers and social workers will often press for confirmation of their suspicions, but even experienced examiners must often take refuge in a neutral report. Remember that charges of sexual assault or child sexual abuse will be keenly fought; experts on both sides are likely to give evidence. When there is uncertainty, the best course is to consult a more experienced colleague, perhaps the local police surgeon or community paediatrician, before embarking on an examination which could have unexpected ramifications.

Patients in custody

Practitioners are not obliged to attend to their patients who have been arrested. In rural areas, force of circumstance may require the police to ask assistance from GPs on a casual basis but, to an increasing extent, appointed police surgeons (or forensic medical examiners) are available to provide medical advice. Police surgeons are specifically mentioned in the Codes of Practice (recently revised) made under PACE as a resource for the custody officer who is responsible for the care of prisoners. At times, remand prisoners have to be accommodated in police cells not equipped to deal with them. These prisoners are moved frequently, leading to an inadequate standard of medical supervision and treatment; there is no proper system for confidential medical records to accompany them for the guidance of doctors who are called subsequently. PACE does not apply in Scotland, but non-statutory provisions with similar effects are in force.

Unless the police surgeon happens to be the prisoner's own GP, NHS scripts may not be issued for those in custody. When a prescription is needed, it must be a private one. Practitioners may be asked by police surgeons for information about current medical history or treatment, and it is to be hoped that all would co-operate with such requests made in the interests of their patient. A high proportion of detainees are on drug treatment for one reason or another (for example, diabetes, epilepsy, angina, asthma and depression) and yet are unable to give an account of these. Many are under the influence of alcohol and a mixture of drugs (some prescribed, some not) which further confuses the clinical picture.

Mental health is frequently a factor raised by custody or arresting officers who witness bizarre behaviour or who have prior knowledge of the accused. Before advising about prisoners to whom the provisions of the Mental Health Act 1983 or the Mental Health (Scotland) Act 1984 apply, police surgeons may seek assistance from GPs. These cases cause much anxiety to doctor and police alike; management in custody is greatly assisted when the relevant history is known. Quite properly, GPs will be reluctant to disclose information to police officers, but in the interests of the unfortunate patients, they should be ready to communicate with their professional colleagues. Caution may, however, need to be exercised if the information could be incriminating.

Only in exceptional circumstances should GPs become involved in matters of clinical forensic medicine as they apply to prisoners, unless acting as police surgeons (*see* below). The general examination of a prisoner has two aims, spelt out by PACE, both requiring specific consent: is the prisoner fit to be detained and is the prisoner fit to be interviewed?

Acting for the defence

A brief description has already been given of the various lesions inflicted in the course of an assault which are likely to present in the surgery. In a proportion of cases patients will allege that the injuries were inflicted by the police during the course of arrest or while the patient was detained. It is the doctor's duty to record the circumstances as related, and the injuries as seen; interpretation is, of course, difficult, especially after the lapse of perhaps several days.

Complaints against the police are directed first of all to the Chief Constable concerned. Each police force has a department which investigates complaints; where there are allegations of ill-treatment, the enquiry is a criminal one, supervised by the Police Complaints Authority (in Scotland, the supervision is by the procurator fiscal). These investigations are rigorous, but cumbersome. The consequence is that many of those who complain feel that their complaint is not being looked at seriously, and are surprised to have a visit many months later to explain the outcome. For the police officers involved, prolonged suspension is often the result, leading to anxiety and depression; even in lesser cases, where suspension is not merited, the symptoms may be sufficiently severe to give rise to sickness absence.

Drink/driving offences

Practitioners may be asked by patients accused of drink/driving offences to act for them, either by immediate examination or by providing a history in exculpation or at least in mitigation. Most convictions are based on measurement of alcohol in a sample of breath using a device installed in the police station. The motorist needs to be properly instructed by the police officer operating the machine before blowing into it (a considerable effort is needed), and may be unable to provide a sufficient sample if frightened, in bronchospasm or without adequate lung volume. No defence based on clinical impression should be offered, but the results of previous lung function testing may be adduced. In the occasional circumstance where blood is taken for analysis, needle phobia has been advanced as a reason for refusal to give permission for venepuncture (a refusal is tantamount to an admission of guilt) but would necessitate relevant history. Without a good deal of background knowledge, it is unsafe to argue about the metabolic removal of alcohol from the blood, and about the likely effect of a particular level. In very few cases does the prosecution depend on clinical examination to secure a conviction. It is unwise to accept a motorist's invitation to attend and examine him in a police station; the doctor called by the police is almost certain to have much greater experience of the necessary procedures, and to be much more familiar with the witness box.

There are two distinct drink driving offences:

1 Driving with excess alcohol (as measured by the alcohol level in breath, blood or urine). In relation to this charge, there is no need to prove any impairment to drive. Either the level of alcohol is above the statutory limit or it is not. (Police forensic laboratories always allow a small leeway of error on the side of the accused).
2 Driving while impaired through alcohol/or drugs. The charge is based on the result of a clinical examination. In relation to this charge, the level of alcohol is not directly relevant. It is the opinion of an experienced Forensic Medical Examiner – which the jury accepts or rejects.

It is possible to be impaired with a blood alcohol below the level (or breath/urine equivalent) of the statutory limit and yet still be clinically not impaired.

Irrespective of the charge a breath sample may be requested at the roadside, using relatively insensitive equipment. The result of this test is only a ground to proceeding to the next stage of investigation (ie the use of the Intoximeter at the police station, the taking of a breath, blood or urine sample or a clinical examination as appropriate).

Information about a history of Parkinsonism, regular prescription of psychoactive drugs or similar factors may assist the motorist and the court. Information of this kind is very helpful in cases of shop-lifting, where there may be a history of depression or some other mitigating factor which, brought to the attention of the authorities, could have the effect of inducing them to drop the prosecution. In recent years, there has been an increasing trend towards the diversion of suitable cases from the courts.

Miscellaneous

In the course of a criminal enquiry, police officers are entitled to scrutinize certain statutory certificates given by medical practitioners. Examples include those given under the Cremation and Abortion Acts. Everyday notes and certificates ranging from the familiar medical statement to endorsement of a passport application are signed with the full moral authority such a signature carries. Questions of medical ethics apart, the doctor who knowingly or carelessly misuses his signature in this way commits a form of perjury.

Patients will often ask for notes excusing them from jury service, attendance as a witness or appearance in the dock. Acute illnesses, such as pneumonia or myocardial infarction or a terminal malignancy might provide an adequate reason in any of these situations. Recovery is to be expected from most illness or injury, and an indication ought to be given when the patient may reasonably be expected to have regained fitness for the particular role. Blanket excuses will not do, nor should the request by the court be taken lightly. Indeed, the certifying doctor is liable to be called to give oral evidence to support his certificate, when he may find himself opposed by a doctor who has been asked by the police or the court to give a second opinion. In Scotland, certificates of this kind must include the formula *attested on soul and conscience* to have validity.

13 Doctors and the courts[1]

Kathleen Allsopp

Responding to solicitors' letters

IT has been said that nothing is more likely to strike fear into the heart of a doctor than a letter from a solicitor. On many occasions the resulting anxiety is so great that doctors prove quite unable to read such letters carefully and to assess what is really required. To misunderstand the point of such approaches can quickly lead to trouble. Before tackling a letter from a solicitor a number of questions must be answered.

Is the letter about a patient who has been treated by the doctor in hospital, the community, private practice or in general practice? Does the letter seek information, clinical records or an opinion? Does the letter indicate on whose behalf it is written?

Consent to release of information

A solicitor should state whether he acts for the patient about whom information is sought or for some other party. If the solicitor does not state this clearly this information must be obtained before responding in detail. If the solicitor states that he acts on behalf of a patient the implication is that the patient consents to his solicitor being given information. Many solicitors, aware of a doctor's over-riding duty of confidentiality, also provide a signed statement from the patient requesting the medical practitioner to release information. If the solicitor states that he does not act for the patient, but for another party, it is imperative that the patient's express consent to the release of information is obtained.

---

[1]Doctors in Scotland should also read Chapter 15 The Differences between Scots and English Law.

What does the solicitor want?

If the doctor is satisfied about consent, the next stage is to decide what the solicitor actually wants. The circumstances in which solicitors may have direct access to patients' clinical records are complex (*see* Chapter 11). In response to a request for the records, to offer a report is inappropriate, although to do so is a common error. The provision of a report as an alternative to disclosure of the records cannot be enforced and has the added disadvantage that by also seeking a fee, a doctor gives quite the wrong impression.

What is the purpose of the report?

If the solicitor is seeking a factual report it is important to establish the grounds for the request.

Factual reports

In many civil matters, unconnected with medical negligence, a solicitor may need evidence of a patient's clinical state in order to demonstrate how an event may have affected his health. It may for instance be necessary to demonstrate that the patient was in good health on a given date in order to show that a specific event had a deleterious effect on his health.

However, it is essential to ensure that the report is only about the patient upon whose behalf the solicitor writes. In matrimonial matters the health and welfare of both parties and their family may be irretrievably bound up in the doctor's mind and indeed often in the doctor's records. Great care should be taken to ensure that any report is restricted to the details about the patient on whose behalf the report is sought, and for whom consent is provided, and no other patient is mentioned (*see* Figure 13.1).

A psychiatrist was consulted by a couple with marital difficulties. Later, having separated, the husband attended again, alone. The wife's solicitors sought a report from the psychiatrist about her but the psychiatrist included details about the husband including information from the later consultations.

On hearing this the husband reported the psychiatrist to the GMC and he was found guilty of serious professional misconduct.

Figure 13.1: Case study

Injuries to patients

Factual reports may be required about incidents involving crime. In such cases, the patient's solicitor may need a precise description of a doctor's findings after an incident such as an assault.

On occasion, solicitors seek reports in connection with allegations of personal injury such as accidents at work or road traffic accidents. Sometimes what is required is a straightforward factual account; but sometimes a solicitor seeks information which would enable his client to claim that whereas the incident was the patient's fault the state in which he now finds himself has been caused by subsequent medical negligence.

Medical negligence

Alternatively, the solicitor may make direct allegations of medical negligence. On receipt of such letters it is important to ascertain whether the solicitor intends to blame the doctor from whom a report is required or whether it is more likely that blame will be attributed to some other party. Before answering such a letter this difference must be clarified. If the solicitor is planning to sue the doctor to whom the letter is addressed, expert advice should be sought before providing a factual report even in what appear to be entirely straightforward circumstances. There are occasions when it may be inappropriate to provide a report at all.

If the report is requested in order to sue another party or another doctor great care should be exercised. It is prudent to ensure that any factual report covers only the activities of the person who prepares it and allows others who may also have been factually involved to make their own statements.

Reports after death

Occasionally a solicitor may require information after a patient's death. Release of some information can have financial implications for the deceased's dependents and care should be taken to ensure that the solicitor requiring the information is properly entitled to receive it. In some circumstances it may be necessary to obtain written consent from the executors.

Testamentary capacity

A doctor may be asked about a patient's testamentary capacity: again it is important to ascertain the reason for the request and to ensure that appropriate consent has been obtained from those empowered to give it. When dealing with a contested will it may be best to prepare a factual account of the doctor's knowledge of the patient at the time when the will was prepared and, given appropriate consent, be prepared to supply the same information to all the parties in dispute, thus avoiding the possibility of appearing to favour one party or another by inadvertently not treating all equally in the terms of the report given.

Expert opinions

A solicitor may write about a patient who has not been under the care of the doctor concerned, asking the doctor to act as an independent expert. No doctor is obliged to undertake such work, but it should be remembered that a patient is as entitled to a second opinion when things may have gone wrong as he is in the clinical context. If senior members of the medical profession who are appropriately experienced and qualified decline to act as experts on behalf of plaintiffs and will only act on behalf of medical defendants, solicitors will be forced to approach those who may be willing but less expert, to the detriment of all concerned. Thus serious consideration should be given to an approach to act as an expert. Sometimes those involved in part of a clinical sequence are asked to act as experts: it is best to avoid being an expert on one's own work or that of one's direct colleagues!

Absurd requests

Occasionally a solicitor's letter is so absurd that it is tempting to ignore it, or to respond with ridicule. It is important to remember that the medical profession's amateur efforts when dabbling in legal matters could be equally amusing to lawyers so a courteous response is indicated at all times (*see* Figure 13.2).

Be courteous

The response to a solicitor's letter sets the tone for subsequent correspondence and probabaly for all future dealings with that solicitor.

A solicitor wrote '. . . during the said operation a very small hole was drilled in our client's left eye. This hole is in the innermost corner of the eye and after the operation is performed the hole should be left uncovered . . . this is to allow substance to escape from the eye. However, when the eye was stitched after the said operation a piece of skin from the nose was attached to the skin of the eye and the said hole was covered. As the substance cannot escape from the eye it seeps underneath into the cheek and . . . is causing the swelling on our client's face'.

A polite but firm response was advised.

Figure 13.2: Case study

Early impressions are important: a response should always be courteous. A solicitor's letter should be acknowledged with an indication that it is receiving prompt attention. This gives the impression of efficiency even if in reality it gives time to seek the all important advice of the defence organization.

Preparing reports

Witnesses can be witnesses to fact, professional witnesses or expert witnesses. In the medical context a factual report given on medical matters becomes the report of a professional witness. A doctor may be a witness of fact when he is merely behaving as a citizen. He might observe a crime being committed or a road traffic accident. Provided that the factual information sought might be given by any citizen this would constitute a factual report. Whenever a doctor gives information about medical matters or a specific patient he cannot escape from being a professional witness. By implication a factual witness or a professional witness has firsthand information to give, whereas an expert witness is an independent commentator without firsthand knowledge of the facts in question.

Preparation of a factual report by a professional witness

1 Give the full name, date of birth and address of the patient as recorded.

2 The doctor should state his own full name and qualifications and his relationship to the patient (e.g. GP).
3 The source of the information should be given (e.g. contemporaneous notes).
4 The report should be dated.
5 An accurate succinct description of the consultation is essential (and much easier from good notes). Care should be taken with details such as the side of the body, the name of the digit and precise description of the site and size of any lesion. Careless mistakes can make a doctor look very silly. If facts cannot be corroborated from contemporaneous records but can be remembered this should be indicated. Although temptations may arise at the time of drafting a medical report the clinical records themselves must never be altered.
6 A factual report may form the basis for subsequent evidence in court. A court appearance may be inescapable if a doctor has firsthand knowledge of the patient and whether or not a report is provided is immaterial in this context. Refusal to provide information, in an effort to avoid a subsequent court appearance, is futile and can earn the criticism of the court.
7 A fee may be payable for a factual report. It is inadvisable to include the note of the fee as part of the report. It should always be a separate submission.

Report of an expert witness

An expert is someone with special expertise based on professional experience and learning and is independent. The request for a doctor to act as an expert should specify whether a report is required on paper or whether an examination of a patient is also needed. A medical expert should note that once the patient has been examined he may himself become a compellable witness since he too, like the factual and professional witness, will now have firsthand knowledge of the patient.

Solicitors' instructions

The solicitor should specify what he wants. It is helpful if he identifies the issues to be addressed. By agreeing to be an expert witness, a doctor should realize that he may be embarking upon a commitment which may last several years, particularly in civil matters which may

within a year in *Naylor* v. *Preston*[2], the Master of the Rolls directed that experts' reports should be disclosed: *'the general rule is that, whilst a party is entitled to privacy in seeking out the "cards" for his hand, once he has put his hand together, the litigation is to be conducted with all the cards face up on the table'*.

Furthermore the recent practice of preparing a bland report and identifying the 'problem areas' in a covering letter to the instructing solicitor has already been identified by the courts as a practice to be discouraged.

Experts may be asked to provide supplementary reports on new information or when other experts have identified new issues which need critical assessment. There is no objection to subsequent reports being provided nor to revision of an original report to include additional comments. However the expert should be wary of having words put in his mouth either by his instructing solicitor or by his fellow experts. The documentation finally provided and described as his own report should indeed be all his own work and express a view he is prepared to stand by.

Witnesses in court

There is much truth in the old adage that a witness should stand up, speak up and shut up. Crucially those who give evidence best as to fact, or as an expert, do it most effectively when well prepared. Although it may be stating the obvious, a witness who treats the court and his legal colleagues with appropriate respect and whose manner, demeanour and dress are that of a fellow professional and who is not afraid to say when he does not know, is less likely to find his time in the witness box stressful.

Giving evidence as a factual/professional witness

One of the most tiresome aspects of giving evidence in criminal trials on minor matters is that there is little warning as to the date, time and place at which testimony must be given. Here much can be achieved by courtesy and goodwill. A genuinely busy practitioner who tries to be available gains more respect than the pretentiously 'grand' doctor.

It is unwise to appear in court to give factual evidence not having refreshed one's memory. It is not expected that all minor details will be committed to memory, but a working familiarity with the sequence of events at issue gives the witness an air of competence and confidence. Whoever is responsible for the attendance of such a witness may not be responsible for reuniting the doctor with his contemporaneous records. This responsibility may fall upon the potential witness. In general practice particularly, patients move and it may take some time to find the relevant general practice notes, so early preparation can be advantageous.

Appearing in court as an expert

In the preparation of much civil litigation, a conference with counsel and the instructing solicitors, the other experts and the plaintiff or defendant is held. It is vital to attend any such conference because that is the opportunity to iron out difficulties in the expert evidence a doctor is expected to give. There is no shame in having second thoughts, or misgivings, provoked by new possibilities raised by fellow experts but the conference is the time for this and not when the expert is in the witness box. The object of the pre-trial conference is not for the expert to be persuaded or rehearsed in the evidence he will give but for counsel to satisfy himself as to the strength of the case and the weight of the experts' opinions.

Counsel will advise as to how much time the expert is needed at the trial and whenever possible the expert should be present at all those times. An expert who only has the time to give evidence on his own behalf and to hear nothing that is said by his fellow experts may not provide counsel with adequate support. If time will be a problem declare this as soon as possible.

The expert who most endears himself to his instructing solicitor has an air of quiet confidence and gives the impression of thoughtfulness and careful consideration. Signs of impatience or imminent loss of temper are inappropriate. Giving convoluted answers leading to further cross-examination endear the expert only to the 'opposing' counsel. It is salutary to remember that in many medical negligence trials the judgement will contain an 'end of term report' on the experts. To be disbelieved by a judge who criticizes an expert's manner, preparation and worst of all expertise may be very distressing (*see* Figure 13.3).

14 European Legislation

Alan Rowe

It is no longer possible, in a book intended for readers in the United Kingdom (UK), to avoid some discussion of international law and, in particular, European Community law. Whilst this chapter will confine itself to Community law it is worth noting that other binding agreements to which the UK is a signatory also have effects on individual citizens. Examples include the Council of Europe Convention for the protection of individuals with regard to automatic processing of personal data (28 January 1981), and the possibility of the UK agreeing to current proposals to include 'trade in services' (including those of doctors) in the General Agreement on Trade in Services (GATT).

Background

The Treaties establishing the European Community comprise the European Coal and Steel Treaty (1951), the Treaty of Rome (1957), the Treaty establishing the European Atomic Energy Community (Euratom 1957), the Single Act (1985) and the Treaty on European Union (Maastrecht 1992). Whilst health is peripheral to the earlier treaties, there have been increasing references to health activities, particularly in the Single Act and in the Treaty on Union.

Nevertheless, health-related products, health professionals and their services are covered by the aims set out in Articles 2 and 3 of the Treaty of Rome. Article 2 refers to promoting '*an accelerated raising of the standard of living*', and Article 3 lists amongst the activities of the Community '*the abolition, as between Member States, of obstacles to freedom of movement for persons, services and capital*', thus including doctors and the provision of healthcare services (*see* Figure 14.1). As this article also calls for the elimination of customs duties and quantitative restrictions on import and export of goods, this includes medicinal products and medical appliances and technical equipment.

The founding fathers of the Community recognized that, for the purposes of free movement of professional persons, mutual recognition of qualifications was necessary, and made provision for this in Article 57(1) of the Treaty of Rome. More importantly, they also recognized that in the case of the medical and allied professions, there was a need for special safeguards, calling for unanimity of decision in the Council of Ministers where implementation of a directive would involve alteration of the principles laid down by law (in any Member State) governing the professions with respect to training and conditions of access to practice by natural persons.

Article 57(2) ' . . . issue directives for the co-ordination of provisions laid down by law in Member States concerning the taking up and pursuit of activities as self-employed persons. Unanimity shall be required on matters which are the subject of legislation in at least one Member State and measures concerned with . . . the conditions governing the exercise of the medical and allied, and pharmaceutical professions in the various Member States.'
Article 57(3) 'In the case of the medical and allied and pharmaceutical professions, the progressive abolition of restrictions shall be dependent upon co-ordination of the conditions for their exercise in the various Member States.'

Figure 14.1:

As the Directives for Doctors were adopted in 1975 and for dentists, midwives, nurses, pharmacists and veterinary surgeons also prior to the Single Act, the clause specifically referring to the medical and allied professions has been omitted from this Act and from the Treaty on European Union.

The Treaty of Rome refers to health in two other articles only. Article 48 provides for a Member State to limit freedom of movement of workers on the grounds of public health (a clause which has always been interpreted by the European Court in a very narrow fashion). Article 117 calls for improved working conditions and an improved standard of living for workers, and Article 118 gives the Commission the task of encouraging closer co-operation between Member States, particularly to promote *'social security, prevention of occupational accidents and diseases, and occupational hygiene'*.

In the Single Act and the Treaty on European Union, further references to health were added to Article 100 (*see* Figure 14.2), which

the United Kingdom), certificates of physical and mental health (required in some countries), and provision for the taking of an oath where this is required.

It is important to recognize that the right to practise in another Member State entails for the migrant the identical rights and obligations to those of a national of the host country. For example, the migrant must abide by the national ethical code. Unlike the United Kingdom, in most other Member States the ethical standards are codified. In some countries this is incorporated in legislation. Although in general ethical principles are identical within the countries of the Community, in some countries there are provisions in the Ethical Code which do not appear in others. It is therefore important that the migrant doctor should familiarize himself with the relevant Code.

Likewise, with widely differing social security systems a doctor must familiarize himself with the details of the national system. Unlike the United Kingdom, in some countries all doctors practise within nationally agreed tariffs as patients are free to consult any physician on any one occasion and to receive reimbursement of the fees. Clearly it is not possible to set out here all the different situations and regulations of the different systems and the reader should seek further information himself either by consulting the national medical association, the competent authority or the Ministry of Health of the host country.

Temporary provision of services (prestation)

The details set out above apply to doctors intending to establish themselves in another Member State. Doctors, in particular private practitioners, may wish from time to time to provide services temporarily for a patient in another country. Article 60 of the Treaty of Rome makes provision for a person who provides service to *temporarily pursue his activity in the State where the service is provided, under the same conditions as are imposed by that State on its own nationals*. Special provisions concerning doctors wishing to temporarily provide services are set out in Article 16 of Directive 75/362/EEC. Most countries require advance notice of intent to provide services, with details as to where and for whom the services are being provided. In urgent cases this information may be provided as soon as possible after the services have been given (Art. 16(2)).

It should also be remembered that in some Member States the law provides that the doctor must ensure 'continuity of care' for the patient and therefore arrangements will have to be made with a resident doctor in the host country to ensure this. Doctors should therefore contact the relevant Competent Authority (in the UK the GMC) if they intend to provide services on a temporary basis. Whilst the phrase 'temporary' has never been defined or legally tested, more than 3 months activity would certainly be regarded as establishment, and French legislation limits 'provision of services' to one person over a 48 hour period.

Drugs and pharmaceutical products

There is a great deal of Community law relating to pharmaceutical products with the objective of achieving harmonization of laws etc. relating to the placing on the market of proprietary medicinal products, based on the criteria of safety, quality and efficacy. They deal not only with manufacture and licensing but also packaging. Unlike the United Kingdom, in most other countries of the Community original pack dispensing has been the norm for many years.

Recently, directives have also dealt with new product licensing and with package inserts. In future, there will be much less difference not only in the labelling of drugs but also in the information provided with the drug pack.

There are however some differences in the national regulation of controlled drugs. In some Member States this can affect the ability of physicians to prescribe these drugs and particularly the quantities that may be prescribed. For example, in palliative care the use of morphine in adequate appropriate dosage may be very difficult for private practitioners.

Liability

Professional liability for negligence exists in all Member States. Unlike the United Kingdom, this risk is normally covered by insurance companies whose activities are strictly limited to underwriting professional risk and do not extend to advising the doctor or defending his professional interest. Membership of a UK defence body however nor-

icians who might contemplate carrying out their own radiological examination when practising in another country it is clearly important to be aware of the provisions of this directive. In the UK this has been incorporated in the relevant radiological protection regulations.

15 The Differences Between Scots and English Law

Helen Philcox

Introduction

IT may seem surprising to many that this chapter is necessary at all, but the fact is that Scottish law, or Scots law as it is known, developed quite independently from English law. To compound matters the Scottish legal system also developed independently and so it too is different, resulting in a confusing variety of terms and legal procedures, particularly in relation to the courts.

The net result is that, even today, the law relating to a GP in Scotland is often very different from that which applies to his English counterpart.

This chapter attempts to outline the main differences in relation to the areas covered elsewhere in this book. Where appropriate, it summarizes what the law is in Scotland and the different legal procedures which apply.

Readers will be relieved to note that in the fields of:

1 Employment law (Chapter 2)
2 European legislation (Chapter 14)
3 The General Medical Council (Chapter 9)

the law is the same north and south of the border. The Mental Health Act and the Mental Health (Scotland) Act, 1960 are similar but not identical.

Negligence (*see* also Chapter 10)

In Scotland the test for medical negligence where deviation from normal practice is alleged, is well established. Three facts require to be proved on the balance of probabilities:

1 It must be proved that there is a usual and normal practise.

An application can also be made under this Section where civil proceedings have already been instituted before the court in question.

Quite separately, once an action is under way, either party can apply to the court for commission and diligence for recovery of documents which is commonly known as a motion to allow a specification of documents. A specification of documents, if allowed by the court, must be served on the person holding the documents referred to in the specification, who may be one of the parties to the action or a third party, unconnected with the action, e.g. a patient's current GP. A special form is also served at the same time and must be completed and returned to the court, together with any documents held.

If a copy of such an order is received, then it is important to read it carefully as only those documents referred to in the specification itself should be disclosed. Disclosure of any information in the medical records which relate to other matters or any third party is not covered by the Specification and remains a breach of the patient's confidentiality.

The form, which usually contains three sections, should be completed by the doctor.

The first section states that all the documents falling within the specification have been produced. The second section states that all the documents in the person's possession have been produced but that he is aware of other documents elsewhere and there is a place to indicate where those documents are. The third part narrates that the person on whom the specification has been served does not have any of the documents specified and does not know where they are.

As the court is likely to keep the records produced in terms of the specification until the case is concluded, it is sensible to take copies of any records produced, as it may be a number of years before the originals are returned.

In Scotland, a patient's records belong to the Secretary of State for Scotland and records themselves are under the control of the Health Board.

The Service Committee and Tribunal Regulations (*see* also Chapter 4)

Although Scotland has its own regulations, (*see* Figure 15.1) these, on the whole, are similar to the regulations which apply in England.

Statutory Instruments	Effective	Title
1974 No.504	01.04.74	The NHS (Service Committees and Tribunals) (Scotland) Regulations 1974
1974 No. 1031	15.07.74	The NHS (Service Committees and Tribunals) (Scotland) Regulations 1974
1988 No. 878 (S.87)	01.06.88	The NHS (Service Committees and Tribunals) (Scotland) Regulation 1988

Figure 15.1: The National Health Service (Service Committees and Tribunals) (Scotland) Regulations 1974 as amended

In Scotland there are no Health Authorities, the Scottish equivalent being a Health Board. Health Boards were set up under the National Health Service (Scotland) Act 1974 Section 2. There are also no Family Health Services Authorities and complaints are heard by Primary Care Divisions or Units set up by each Health Board.

In terms of the Act, Health Boards are required to keep a list of all GP's who are contracted to provide services within the Board's own particular area. Any complaint about a GP must be made to the general manager of the appropriate Board on whose list the name of the GP is entered.

Normally, any patient making a complaint must do so in writing and the complaint must relate to something which is potentially a breach of the terms of the GP's contract with the Health Board i.e. his Terms of Service.

The normal time limit for making a complaint is 6 weeks from the date of the matter giving rise to the complaint. A late complaint can still be considered but the Service Committee must be satisfied that the failure to make the complaint in time was due to a good reason, such as illness. If the Board is satisfied of this it has the power to allow a complaint outwith the 6 week period, up to a period of 2 months of the matter coming to the complainer's notice.

Any further extension of the time limit depends on the Committee obtaining the consent of the GP or, if he refuses to give his consent, of the Secretary of State for Scotland.

If the time limits are not complied with or dispensed with or the Secretary of State's consent is not obtained, it is incompetent for a Service Committee to deal with the case.

distinct from the individual partners. A firm can sue or be sued separately (1890 Act, Section 4(2)).

2 In relation to contracts, in Scotland the individual partners in a firm are liable not only jointly, but also severally, for any debts incurred or obligations undertaken by the firm. This means that anyone who sues the firm has the option of suing a particular partner or several of the partners for the whole sum which they allege is due. It is then up to the individual partner or partners concerned to pursue their fellow partners for the proportionate share due by each of them (1890 Act, Section 9).

3 In relation to wrongs, that is actions relating to alleged negligence by one or more of the partners, liability is again joint and several (1890 Act, Section 12).

4 Section 23 of the 1890 Act relates to proceedings against partnership property for a partner's separate judgment debt. This Section does not apply to Scotland.

5 Section 47 of the Act provides that nothing in the Act affects the Scottish law of bankruptcy.

6 Separately, the National Health Service (Scotland) Act 1978, Section 35 prohibits the sale of goodwill in relation to medical partnerships.

7 Partnership agreements often include a clause which seeks to limit the right of a retired partner to practise as a GP in the vicinity, normally for a fixed period. In England these are known as binding out clauses but in Scotland they are known as restrictive covenant clauses.

Dealing with death (*see* also Chapter 6)

In Scotland there is no coroner and no coroner's inquest. The Scottish equivalent is the procurator fiscal who is a lawyer, and a fatal accident inquiry. The present system was set up under the Fatal Accident and Sudden Deaths Inquiry (Scotland) Act 1976.

This Act details the purposes of a fatal accident inquiry, the way in which it is to be conducted and also the basic machinery for preliminary investigations which are carried out by the procurator fiscals' department.

Any sudden death should be reported to the procurator fiscal who will usually carry out a preliminary investigation into the matter. He will also investigate any death which occurs in circumstances likely to be of public interest or concern or if the deceased's relatives press for a public inquiry.

In carrying out an investigation, the fiscal will take statements from all medical staff involved in the treatment of the patient prior to death. This is often the first indication to a GP that a fatal accident inquiry may take place.

Most doctors involved in an inquiry are professional witnesses as to fact. This means that any questions they are asked will normally relate to their own involvement in that particular case.

Sometimes the fiscal will want a doctor not involved in the deceased's treatment to appear as an independent expert witness and, if so, the fiscal will make this clear from the beginning and ask for the doctor's opinion about the case.

Once statements have been obtained from everyone involved in the case, the fiscal will send the papers to the Crown Office in Edinburgh where a decision is taken whether to hold a fatal accident inquiry. If a death occurs during the course of employment, or in custody, an inquiry is compulsory. Otherwise, it is at the discretion of the Crown Office and procurator fiscal.

The inquiry itself is not a trial but is a fact-finding inquiry held in the Sheriff Court for the district in which the death occurred. The fiscal presents the case to the court and leads all the witnesses. He asks them questions first. Anyone with an interest in the inquiry can ask to be legally represented at it and this is usually allowed. Legal representatives of the family or of doctors appearing at the inquiry are entitled to ask questions of any of the witnesses after the procurator fiscal. At the end of all the evidence, the sheriff is required to make a decision known as a determination. In terms of Section 6(1) of the 1976 Act his determination must state where and when the death or any accident resulting in the death took place and the cause or causes of death. The sheriff is empowered to go on to make a finding about any reasonable precautions which might have prevented the death or any accident resulting in the death. The sheriff can also make a finding in his determination about any defect in any system which he considers contributed to the death or any other facts he thinks relevant to the circumstances of the death.

When a GP is requested by the fiscal to attend an inquiry he will receive a formal court citation which is delivered by two policemen. At the inquiry itself a shorthand writer will be present to write down everything that is said by witnesses and lawyers.

If a party has made out a relevant case, or if he amends his case, the action will then proceed to proof (trial). This is a full hearing of the case where evidence is led on behalf of both parties including expert evidence. Very few actions of medical negligence actually come to proof and it is usually cases where there is a genuine difference of expert opinion which come before a court.

At the end of the proof the judge has to consider all of the evidence he has heard, including the expert evidence and he will make findings of fact on the basis of which he will decide, on the balance of probabilities, in favour of one or other party to the action.

Sheriff Court

The Sheriff Court has the power to deal exclusively with actions up to a value of £1500. It can also deal with actions where the sum sued for is greater than £1500. To some extent, its remit overlaps that of the Court of Session. There are a number of Sheriff Courts in Scotland and each deals with a specific geographical area.

The type of action raised in the Sheriff Court depends on the amount of damages sought.

Small claims summons. This document must be used if the damages sought are less than £750. In this type of action a simplified procedure is used, but the small claims summons must identify the parties to the action, set out the amount sued for and have attached to it a statement of claim detailing the pursuer's case, including any allegations of negligence.

Summary cause summons. This document must be used if the damages sought are between £750 and £1500. The information in the summons is effectively the same as that which requires to be set out in a small claims summons. Again, there is a particular procedure which must be followed in this type of action.

Initial writ. This document must be used if the damages sought are more than £1,500.

In both summary cause procedure and small claims procedure, the court will initially fix a date which is known as a return day by which time a defender must notify the court if he intends to defend the action or if the claim is admitted. If he does nothing, the pursuer may apply to the court for decree together with expenses.

If the defender advises the court he intends to defend the action by returning a particular form, then he must appear in court 1 week after the return day. This appearance is called a preliminary hearing in small claims procedure and calling date in summary cause procedure. When the defender appears in court he must notify the court of his defence which is noted on the summons. A further hearing is fixed and this is known as a full hearing in the case of a small claim or a proof if it is a summary cause action. At both, evidence is led from witnesses as to fact and expert witnesses before the judge, who is known as a sheriff, after which he will consider the case and issue a decision, which is called a judgement. This sets out the judge's findings in fact and his decision as to which party has proved his case on the balance of probabilities.